SUGAR NATION

SUGAR NATION

THE HIDDEN TRUTH BEHIND
AMERICA'S DEADLIEST HABIT AND
THE SIMPLE WAY TO BEAT IT

JEFF O'CONNELL

HYPERION

NEW YORK

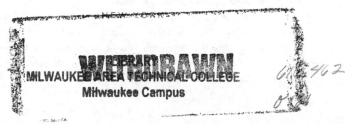

Library of Congress Cataloging-in-Publication Data

O'Connell, Jeff.
Sugar nation : the hidden truth behind America's deadliest habit and the simple way to beat it / Jeff O'Connell.
p. cm.
Includes index.
ISBN 978-1-4013-2344-8
1. Non-insulin-dependent diabetes—Popular works.   2. Diabetes—United States.
3. O'Connell, Jeff—Health.   4. Prediabetic state—Patients—
United States—Biography.   I. Title.
RC662.18.O36 2010
616.4'62—dc22
2010031227

Hyperion books are available for special promotions, premiums, or corporate training. For details contact the HarperCollins Special Markets Department in the New York office at 212-207-7528, fax 212-207-7222, or email spsales@harpercollins.com.

Book design by Chris Welch

FIRST EDITION

10 9 8 7 6 5 4 3

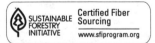

THIS LABEL APPLIES TO TEXT STOCK

We try to produce the most beautiful books possible, and we are also extremely concerned about the impact of our manufacturing process on the forests of the world and the environment as a whole. Accordingly, we've made sure that all of the paper we use has been certified as coming from forests that are managed, to ensure the protection of the people and wildlife dependent upon them.

For Joe Weider

We shape our tools and then our tools shape us.

—*Marshall McLuhan*

CONTENTS

SUGAR NATION

INTRODUCTION

Sugar and temptation have enjoyed a long and colorful history, since the Beginning. Adam and Eve were lounging around blissfully in the Garden of Eden when Eve offered Adam an apple—fructose and glucose, surrounded by some fiber. Tempted, Adam took a bite. There's no way to know for certain, but chances are that he liked this new sensation very much. After all, sugar is sweet, and sweet is good.

Were they here today, Eve could sabotage Adam just as easily by taking him to a drive-through, ordering a number three, and handing him a bag filled with a double cheeseburger and fries, along with an up-sized soda. And if Adam were tempted by the sweet taste and convenience, he'd probably end up with a gut, high triglycerides, and type 2 diabetes.

Fast-forward from the days of "Let There Be Light." Sugarcane grows for the first time in New Guinea, a Polynesian island. Enterprising merchants carry the plant along trade routes to China and India, where in 500 B.C., enterprising scientists notice that when boiled, sugarcane leaves behind a sort of fairy dust. Workdays don't yet begin with an espresso

1

macchiato—alas, no Starbucks yet—but it doesn't take long for tongues to be tantalized by the addition of those tiny crystals to various foods and beverages. That original sugar was actually pretty healthy, containing protein, fiber, and other nutrients.

Sugar reaches Europe in the Middle Ages, further firing up the Crusaders. Columbus takes some sugarcane along with him to the New World, where, in another five hundred years or so, it will prove deadlier than guns or germs. The first sugarcane on U.S. shores is planted in Louisiana in the mid-eighteenth century. Over time, our appetite for all things sweet grows, and food scientists learn clever new ways to feed an ever-growing addiction, to the tune of 160 pounds of sugar a year. That's how much the average American now consumes.

Sugar has gone from expensive to cheap, from healthy to unhealthy. That's because most of its redeeming value has been processed away. Sugar is now dense in energy, but those calories are largely empty.

Along with sweetening food, sugar also helps other calories generate longer shelf lives. It preserves, à la salt. Sprinkle some on a slab of meat hanging from the rafters of Grandpa Jed's barn, or on some lunch meat shrink-wrapped for the supermarket, and those foods won't spoil as fast. If nothing else, you see, sugar has staying power.

Like poor Adam, I never knew what hit me. Up until the fall of 2006, I ate and drank a lot of sugar, largely unaware of type 2 diabetes, because only the old and the overweight need worry about it, I thought. How wrong I was. My ignorance is inexcusable, given that I wrote for a magazine called *Men's Health*, but it also goes a long way toward explaining why the disease has spread across America with the persistence of a glacier and the devastation of a wildfire. As it stands, one in three American adults has type 2 diabetes or its preamble, prediabetes. Remarkably, one in four diabetics is in the dark about his or her condition. One of them might be you.

If you are, this book will shine a bright light on the enemy lurking within. Please, don't fear that revelation. It's what you do next that matters the most. But the time to start is now. Medical self-awareness, in fact, could end up saving your life. You don't have to be diabetic to benefit from controlling your blood sugar, because everyone can use the know-how in this book to boost their energy, sharpen their focus, and live longer and more healthfully.

Diabetes has snuck up on America because insulin resistance, its root cause, sneaks up on Americans. It's the invisible cause of an invisible disease. By the time someone learns they're prediabetic, insulin resistance is already in charge, and probably has been for many years. Such stealth explains why no one—young or old, thin or overweight, man or woman—should assume they're safe from this deadly disease. Diabetes snuck up on me too, because I was neither old nor overweight, and because I was ignorant of my own family history. When I knew the truth, I was stunned, and dazed, and a little frightened. Because I didn't know any better.

I didn't know, for example, that the chemicals released by sugar consumption travel the same brain pathways that heroin does, and that when we're stressed, or sad, the foods that can produce this feeling exert a magnetic pull.

I didn't know that the best way to lose weight and keep it off is to do the exact opposite of what the majority of mainstream weight-loss experts recommend.

I didn't know that when you receive your first diabetes drug prescription, that's just the starter kit, and no one knows that better than the doctors and drug makers.

I didn't know that blood sugar volatility is a dangerously overlooked risk factor for cardiovascular disease, and that most diabetes tests don't measure it.

I didn't know that most physicians don't do a very good job of counseling their patients on lifestyle decisions, particularly when it comes to diet and physical activity.

I didn't know that when you develop insulin resistance and neglect it, the condition inevitably worsens. Whether the statistical threshold to diabetes is crossed in three months or three years, the toll is a heavy one indeed. I've seen it for myself.

What I did know? That my limbs, heart, and kidneys were worth a hell of a lot more to me than hamburger buns, French fries, and glazed doughnuts. So I changed my ways with a vengeance. It began with a primal survival urge, suddenly awoken. But I was also fueled by curiosity, about how this disease works and why it's so deadly; and anger, that type 2 diabetes has this aura of inexorability, when it is in fact preventable and manageable, if not reversible. I became determined not to become one of the disease's victims, and to inform others while waging my own personal battle.

Now, of course, I know much more than that. My four-year diabetes journey only matters as a telescope for viewing the story that matters: the full extent of our national sugar sickness. Sugar gave rise to the slave trade; now sugar has enslaved us. As a result, America's most preventable disease, type 2 diabetes, has taken over instead. It's bad enough that the American disease of the twenty-first century is man-made, but its ascent to Public Health Enemy Number One represents a collective failure breathtaking in more ways than one.

Many people who are fighting a disease sometimes are thankful for the perspective gained from learning how fleeting life can be. They appreciate things more. I understand that. But when I say that prediabetes gave me a new lease on life, take those words literally. I'm a much better person now than I was when I learned of my own blood-sugar meltdown. I'm healthier, fitter, more focused, and more energized than I ever was before.

Make no mistake about it. Diabetes is an awful disease. Should it gain the upper hand, death itself can seem a welcome reprieve. But if you recognize the warning signs early enough and take corrective action, you'll do more than beat this disease. You'll also transform your life.

First, though, you need a plan of action. Unfortunately the industry that has mushroomed around type 2 diabetes measures success in approvals for new drugs, revenue earned, and money raised, not in suffering avoided or lives saved. Whether I was sitting in an exam room with my doctor, visiting the largest diabetes conferences in the world, reading journal articles, or interviewing experts at major universities, I kept coming back to the same realization over and over again. To avoid a long and torturous demise at the hands of diabetes, I'd have to hit the road to figure out this thing on my own.

You shouldn't have to do that.

1

GROUND ZERO

DIABETES IN THE DELTA

Deep in the heart of the Mississippi delta, the sick fill a waiting room in the Mallory Community Health Center. Children skip among the swollen feet of middle-aged women, dodge the canes of old men, and bounce off the ample girth of their young diabetic mothers. I'm being led to a back office, and one patient remains between the door and me. He looks to be between forty and fifty years old. His arms are toned from the sort of repetitive, slow-twitch muscle work normally handled by the legs. I've seen his gaze before, in the eyes of someone whose body has been taken apart and whose spirit has vacated the premises. Looking down, I see that his legs end where they should begin, at the hips. Stumps rest on a wheelchair seat.

In Lexington, Mississippi, the health clinics are flooded with victims of type 2 diabetes. So are the retail stores, sandwich shops, banks, used-tire stores, courthouses, churches, and graveyards. In the United States, one in every ten adults suffers from this disease, which is the end result of a lifestyle that includes too many carbohydrates and other calories and too little physical activity. The number of type 2s falls closer to one in seven in Holmes County, of which Lexington is the county seat. Many diabetics have no clue they're even sick, especially in an area such as this, where high school graduation rates are low, and where many are on Medicare or are uninsured. If the delta's blues greats of yore were alive today, type 2 diabetes would be the hellhound on their trail.

Inside a back office, I ask Reginald Rigsby, M.D., who is one of the clinic's doctors, how many of the patients at this federally funded clinic are diabetics. Forty percent, is his estimate, and he ticks off risk factors: "Obesity, genetic predisposition, poor diet, lack of exercise, smoking, drinking—you name it," he says. I ask the doctor if he becomes frustrated when his warnings of amputations and blindness fall on deaf ears. "I used to take it home with me, but I had to let go a long time ago," he says with a shrug. "I'm just one man in a sea of disparity." It's a fitting image, since type 2 diabetes preys most often on those who are the most economically disadvantaged.

Before my tour ends, I peek inside the clinic's exercise room, arrayed with an assortment of free weights and cardio equipment. Where combating diabetes is concerned, lifestyle changes such as exercising and calorie-and-carb cutting beat drug therapies every time there's a face-off in clinical trials. The more helpful lifestyle changes that diabetics make, the greater the victory. It's no contest, in fact.

So imagine if you were diagnosed with cancer and, in the midst of the terror and panic, the doctor offered you a deal: "Change your diet and exercise, and I can virtually guarantee your survival." It's an offer that would be hard to resist, right? You might even start doing jumping jacks right there in the doc's office, after collapsing to your knees in gratitude.

Unfortunately, the treadmills here at the clinic sit idle. The waiting room is packed and the parking lot is full—the patients don't walk here—but the workout room is empty save for my tour guide and me. That's the thing. We know exactly what causes this disease, and we know how to prevent it, even to reverse it. We have the tools at our disposal.

So why aren't we using them?

·   ·   ·

HOLMES COUNTY IS one of the front lines of America's war with
diabetes, only you would think an armistice was already in place, given
the number of white flags being waved. But at least one man hasn't
given up; he wants to defeat diabetes, not surrender.

Thirty minutes before Harsh Doshi, M.D., had brought me to the
clinic, I spied him standing in his doorway, gesturing welcome in his
shirt and tie. He yelled for me to park on the front lawn, next to his
own beat-up Toyota Corolla. His business attire is neat, but the doctor's house appears to have been ransacked, perhaps because he shares
it with his sixteen-year-old son. Dr. Doshi tells me coffee is brewing,
and the kitchen I enter in search of it is even more disheveled than the
living room. Stacks of pots and pans teeter on rotting countertops lined
with old newspapers. Dishes, clean and dirty, are everywhere. A plastic
cutting board is dangerously close to a stove burner. The only sign that
a doctor might live here is the Vioxx promo magnet stuck on the rusted-
out refrigerator door. Clearly, this is a man with more on his plate than
cleaning house.

Dr. Doshi enters, makes himself a bowl of Cheerios, and leads me
out to the front porch, where we sit ten feet apart on opposite hanging
benches. A young boy from the neighborhood walks up, sits down beside me, looks up, and gently rocks our swing. Foliage grows crazily
throughout the region, I've noticed, but I can't draw my gaze from the
overgrowth across the street, so untamed that it takes me a while to dis-
cern a house buried underneath. Even a mangy dog seems bewildered
as it emerges from the thicket.

I start by asking Dr. Doshi, fifty-two, where he's from. He says, "Essentially, life narrows down to *hu-man-ity*." He will begin many answers
with ponderous non sequiturs like that one; nonetheless, a less likely or
better guide to take me through the Mississippi delta, I can't imagine.
His mother was a linguistics professor and his father a stockbroker in India, his native land. His own calling was medicine, and after a brief stint
teaching in a Saudi Arabia health care center, he did a year's residency in
Toledo, Ohio, then three additional years of residency in internal medicine at Oakwood Hospital & Medical Center in Dearborn, Michigan.

In order to convert his J-1 Exchange Visitor Visa into a green card and remain with his U.S.-born son, who was then a year old, he was required to work for two years in a rural area of the United States. So without knowing a soul down in the delta, he moved there in 1994, becoming the first physician to work at Mallory, in a health clinic being started by an MIT-trained nutrition specialist with the aid of a federal grant. Dr. Doshi was assigned chronic disease management, which in an area like this is akin to learning surgery in a war zone. Fifteen years later, long after he could have left the region for an easier practice and Friday afternoons on the links, he remains here, a proud U.S. citizen dedicated to caring for those who need him the most.

"I've fallen in love with these people, and I can see their suffering through my heart," he tells me. "As a physician, if I can't understand your suffering, I cannot solve your problem. If I reflect on my own life, what good did I do? If I can say that I have crossed the barrier to love the people, and care for them, without realizing who they are or not, focusing on their minds, bodies, spirits, then I have lived my life." He concludes such statements by cocking his head and widening his eyes, as if he's delivered a soliloquy to the boy and me.

He appreciates me coming to this place and finding him, but he also challenges my motivations. I explain that my father is dying from diabetes, and that I've been informed that the same killer is after me now. "You had a personal experience which prompted you to take an interest and follow it further," he says. "But do you *have* to put your hand in the *fire* to feel how it burns? That is a question that you must ask yourself: Can I be so sensitive as to understand the suffering of other human beings?"

I had already asked myself that question, actually. I thought back to my skepticism regarding the motives of philanthropists who would donate some princely sum to build a new hospital wing in their name, dedicated to curing whatever disease had stricken them or a loved one. *That disease was there before you ever got it*, I would think. *That's your ego responding to a tragedy, not your heart*. Now, standing in their shoes, in a sense, I wondered if my motives were any less conflicted and impure. For a writer like me, maybe a byline was the equivalent of a name stenciled on the facade of a building.

Regardless, the problem needs solving. Few regions have hosted more human suffering than this one, and type 2 diabetes has joined poverty and obesity on a long list of slave masters. My Indian guide takes me from the Mallory clinic in Lexington to another one in nearby Tchula. This town was a regular stop along the juke-joint circuit covered by post–World War II–era blues legends such as Elmore James, but "things ain't what they used to be," to quote one of his classics. I follow a cloud of dust up an unpaved driveway filled with small craters; the next thing I know, Dr. Doshi is wrestling with his lab coat while hurrying inside.

I interview him in between his meetings with patients, most of them diabetics. Anytime he leaves his office for a consultation, the urgency of his lecture can be heard through the walls. After returning, he sits behind his desk, and his tone becomes more measured. "From the physician's point of view, treating diabetes and its comorbidities is time-consuming and complex," he says. "You cannot solve it in a day or two. These are long-term situations."

While he fields a phone call, I pick up a leaflet from the table next to me in his office: *What Is Type 2 Diabetes?* In simple language, it explains how something called insulin resistance leads to diabetes. There are even diagrams resembling those found in a newsstand health magazine. Flipping it over, I see diabetes treatments presented as a series of simple steps: "Diet and exercise," "Add diabetes pill(s)," "Add basal insulin," "Add mealtime (bolus) insulin." Drugs aren't treated as a last resort. They're all part of the natural progression. What you can't do, pills and shots presumably can. And isn't taking a pill much easier than reengineering the way you lead your life?

"Remember, insulin is only a part of treating diabetes," the brochure instructs. "Following a meal plan, staying active, regularly checking your blood sugar levels, and taking all diabetes medications as prescribed are also important steps." Not surprisingly, Sanofi-Aventis, a pharmaceutical giant that manufactures diabetes drugs, produced this "educational" material.

· · ·

I MEET SEVERAL of Dr. Doshi's patients. One of them, Ruth Tolbert, is a sixty-six-year-old African-American who found out she was a type 2 diabetic in 2005. One of fourteen children whose parents were also type 2s, she always felt that diabetes was her destiny. "I was waiting till it got to me," she says. She felt helpless; but even though she was a career nurse, she didn't know that her diet could help prevent diabetes. "Now I do, but it's too late," she says. "People with a family history should eat like a diabetic starting off from when they're tiny tots. I tell my grandkids to eat like they're diabetic already, and they'll have no problems later on." First, though, they need to know what a healthy diabetic diet actually looks like on the plate.

Ruth thought she was eating healthfully most of her adult life until a book she read one day told her otherwise. She stayed active, walking not only to get from one place to another but also for its own sake. But she gladly would have changed other habits—including eliminating potatoes with her steak and vegetables, cutting out high-sugar desserts—had she only known that they were sabotaging her well-intentioned efforts in other areas.

Type 2 diabetes doesn't swarm over immune defenses the way cancer does. It decommissions the foes capable of warding it off, one by one, until it can act unchecked. Outsmarting the disease means not only managing your blood sugar but also sidestepping complications such as heart disease, kidney shutdown, nerve damage, and amputations. Ruth's battle has become harder, she says, since she suffered a stroke. The damage inflicted by high blood sugar on blood vessels in the brain doubles the risk of having one of these attacks. She speaks softly and deliberately, but the only time her face turns sad is when she reveals that her husband won't take her fishing anymore. She has trouble boarding the boat because of stroke-related balance and strength challenges. She needs a cane, and her right foot is balky and prone to swelling.

Now that she knows what to do, she goes the extra mile—fifty-five of them, in fact. That's how far she drives from Tchula to Jackson to purchase Ezekiel 4:9 bread, a high-fiber food whose blood sugar effects are benign, and brown rice instead of the white rice that's on sale in Lexington's grocery stores. "The food is terrible around here," she says.

"We don't have good markets or food stores, and the restaurants are really bad. They give you two starches on your plate." One reason she came here today was to score a pass to the exercise room I had seen earlier at the Lexington health center. But she worries that she's losing the fight, periodically casting a nervous glance down at that ailing foot of hers.

After fifteen minutes of conversation, she confides a secret: "Don't tell Dr. Doshi, but I stopped taking the metformin about three months ago. I take a blood sugar tea from the health food store every day instead. It keeps my blood sugar down and makes me feel better than the pill does. The metformin made me very hungry. At lunchtime, I'd be starving. I just couldn't stand it anymore." It's an interesting anecdote, since the drug is purported to suppress appetite.

A common refrain among health care givers here in Holmes County is that residents don't have ready access to foods such as fresh produce, confirming Ruth Tolbert's personal experience. But I drive to lunch with Dr. Doshi through the richest farmland I've ever beheld, with rivers carving their way through lush, green fields. I wonder how people could be chronically malnourished in what appears to be an agricultural Shangri-la. They're surrounded by fresh produce that doesn't belong to them and is headed elsewhere, as it turns out. So they eat what they can afford, which isn't much.

The median household income in Holmes County is $23,369. Worrying about type 2 diabetes down the road often takes a backseat to feeding hungry mouths that night. "For many of the people who live here, it's far cheaper to live off McDonald's or Popeyes or lots of pastas and white rice—carbs and unhealthy fats—than to eat healthfully," says Gabriel I. Uwaifo, M.D., associate professor at the University of Mississippi Medical Center in Jackson.

This diabetes divide isn't backwater regions versus the big city. The urban and suburban poor are just as diabetes-prone as the rural poor. The bonds between the disease and poverty are interwoven at very fine scales of geographic resolution throughout the country. At the University of Washington's Center for Public Health Nutrition, researchers use census tract data, which is more specific than ZIP codes, to map obesity and diabetes. Block by block, those conditions overlay poverty. If you took a hypothetical affluent neighborhood and placed it side by side with a poor one, diabetes rates in the poor neighborhood would predictably exceed rates on the affluent street by a widening margin.

"You can't say that people with a given genetic predisposition up and moved to a given census tract down by I-5," says the center's director, Adam Drewnowski, Ph.D., a leading expert in the field. "This disease is environmental and economic. Unless we do something about our social disparities, we're toast as a nation when it comes to type 2 diabetes."

For lunch at Los Molcajetes in nearby Flora, Dr. Doshi and I are joined by his girlfriend, Julie, a Mississippi native whose wide body squishes his into one-third of their side of the booth. They met when she was working in housekeeping at one of the clinics; eleven years later, they remain together.

"When it comes to diabetes, access to health care is key," says Dr. Doshi after a few bites. "But the patient needs to desire the care. Diabetes is only one manifestation of not only a medical problem but also a behavioral problem. Poor diet, lack of exercise, stress—so many things go hand in hand. If you don't give them treatment, eventually they will become sicker or die. You pay a greater price later on to the suffering of our own people than we can do by taking corrective measures ahead of time." That's an understatement. The key to solving this public health crisis lies with prevention, or, failing that, early detection and swift lifestyle change.

Dr. Doshi strikes me as having the heart and soul of a modern-day Hippocrates. Still, despite his passion, what he can't tell me is exactly *how* diabetics should diet to lose weight or *how* they should exercise or *how* they should reduce their stress levels. Like most doctors, probably like your doctor, he follows the guidelines issued by the American Diabetes Association (ADA). It's the only tool he has, but it's not the best one.

The ADA's stated mission is "to prevent and cure diabetes and to improve the lives of all people affected by diabetes." I'm not convinced that this mission has been met, that those guidelines are serving us as they should. Beyond that—well, patients can always rely on one of those brochures from drug companies, among the ADA's biggest benefactors. At every juncture, the leading diabetes authorities suggest that patients can't or won't make the necessary lifestyle changes. Their alternative is a reliance on drug after drug to manage what becomes a long, painful, complications-riddled demise. When they could just cure the disease.

THE ADA AND many doctors pay only lip service to lifestyle change, so people forgo an ounce of prevention in favor of pound after pound of cure. Sure, patients are handed a pamphlet with their prescriptions telling them that diet and exercise would, in fact, help. But the unspoken assumption is that the patient will never stick with the lifestyle program.

"Very few people participate in dietary changes and physical activity, so you end up with patients not taking care of their diabetes," says Larry C. Deeb, M.D., an endocrinologist and ADA past president for medicine and science. "My take is, let me give you a prescription. No rule says I can't take you off the medicine later."

Swallowing a pill is easier than swallowing that logic. If only we invested as much effort honing message delivery as we do perfecting drug delivery. Hearing many physicians discuss lifestyle change as an alternative to diabetes drugs reminds me of the Pledge of Allegiance or a religious hymn being repeated only as a matter of habit. These can be powerful messages, but not when they're delivered with the hollowness of elevator music. How persuasive can any argument in favor of lifestyle change be when moments later the same doctor is talking up prescription drugs, per the ADA guidelines?

Back in early 2002, the medical world was stunned when a combination of lifestyle changes (dietary adjustments, exercise, and the resulting weight loss) reduced diabetes incidence by 58 percent in the Diabetes Prevention Program, a major multicenter clinical research study. The superstar of type 2 diabetes drugs, metformin, reduced it by only 31 percent. Problem solved, you might think.

"That was now *eight* years ago," says Steven N. Blair, P.E.D., professor of exercise science at the University of South Carolina. "How has that not transformed medical practice? It's just astonishing. Lifestyle change is twice as effective and costs much less. We've got to prevent diabetes, and that's how you do it."

The fate of those with high blood sugar and diabetes needn't be the foregone conclusion portrayed in doctors' offices, in the media, and elsewhere in our country. Unlike cancer, or multiple sclerosis, or Alzheimer's, the solution for type 2 diabetes is crystal clear. This disease can be sent packing using any number of strategies and techniques, none of which requires a drug prescription.

People just need to be told what they are.

NEW ORLEANS, THAT symbol of bungled disaster relief, is a fitting backdrop for the ADA's sixty-ninth annual meeting in early June 2009. Metabolic gurus from around the world have convened at the city's convention center to fight the disease; this is their Super Bowl, and the scale is similarly epic. On TV monitors hanging above the hallways, anchors—or actors playing anchors—bleat the latest diabetes breakthroughs, as if CNN were delivering a news flash. In all, fifteen thousand people, thirteen thousand of them researchers and health care professionals, will attend. Since its inception, the ADA has invested more than $450 million and provided funding for more than four thousand research projects. When I pick up my press credentials, the summary of research abstracts I'm handed is so hefty that I wonder if the diabetics in attendance shouldn't just use it as a dumbbell.

Experts are on hand to discuss the use of stem cells to grow new insulin-producing cells in the pancreas. Bariatric surgeons will explain how they can tie up an obese diabetic's stomach like a carnival balloon for up to $26,000 a pop, procedures called gastric bypass and gastric banding. In 2008, 220,000 of the desperately overweight undertook such bariatric surgeries in the United States alone. Epidemiological studies are reviewed, clinical trials updated, and panels convened to discuss everyone from the diabetic athlete to students with diabetes to pregnant women with gestational diabetes, a form of the disease that usually leaves once the baby arrives.

Later that day, a block away from the convention center, the ADA conference's reception is under way. The bar is crowded, and behind it, a line snakes past a long buffet. Holly Clegg, the author of *Holly Clegg's trim&Terrific Diabetic Cooking*, has prepared the cuisine for the reception at the ADA's behest. The chicken lettuce wraps and chicken rosemary strips would be compatible with my low-carb diet, but the pasta jambalaya and berry tiramisu—with 51 and 23 carb grams per serving, respectively—wouldn't. I aim to consume 80 or fewer grams of carbs (excluding fiber) *a day* to keep prediabetes at bay.

Low-carb experts have convinced me this amount can keep my brain and body functional and healthy, especially since I choose whole food sources of mostly complex carbs with lots of fiber. I might have half a cup of oatmeal with breakfast, some edamame with lunch, an apple, and broccoli at dinner—not a Coke before bed. Bear in mind that, following the ADA's lead, health organizations around the globe are telling diabetics *never* to consume fewer than 130 carb grams a day. They claim even that amount is extremely low, and that anything below that threshold literally will starve the brain and central nervous system. But after four years eating amounts well below their lower limit, my mind is sharp. My body feels great. I can power through forty-five-minute daily workouts. The only thing that seems helpless to function under these conditions, actually, is diabetes.

The ingredient lists for the six dishes being served at the reception include reduced-fat or fat-free versions of dressings, broths, cream cheese, whipped topping, yogurt, and mayonnaise. It strikes me as a strange fixation, this fat phobia among mainstream weight-loss and diabetes experts. After all, fat has virtually no impact on blood sugar. The same can't be said of the carbs substituted to make those products low-fat, or fat-free, or "light." Even the most respected voices on the topic of diabetes are missing the point when it comes to diet, replacing the scapegoat, dietary fat, with the true culprit, carbs. So instead of eating the meals prepared on behalf of the ADA, which aren't on my diet, I head to Bourbon Street.

The progression of diabetes pits the body against the brain, which must impose the discipline needed to control the disease: *Don't* do this.

Don't eat that. And please, don't even *consider* drinking that. What, are you crazy? Those edicts are easy to ignore when floating in a stream of neon, incense, laughter, and blaring trumpets on a Friday night. I could take my pick—temptations lurk everywhere here. Next to one cabaret fronted by two nearly naked young women, a sign reads BIG ASS BEERS TO GO. I'm not sure if that refers to the size of the drink or its effect on the drinker. While mulling that, I spy what looks like a voodoo priestess peering my way from a fortune-teller's storefront. And Bourbon Street could be renamed for the daiquiri, so freely do these spirits flow, sweetened with 2 grams of sugar per fluid ounce. That's 20 grams of carbs in a ten-ounce drink.

A beer or daiquiri could help wash down the sandwich that is synonymous with this party town. The po' boy, it's called, and Subway spokesman Jared Fogle would faint at the very sight of one. French bread is cut in half, deep-fried, and then heaped with a filling such as fried shrimp. For a diabetic, the problem isn't the deep-frying, or the shrimp, or the dressings, which can include lettuce, tomato, pickles, mustard, mayonnaise, and onions. The problem is the French bread and the breading overlaying the shrimp. All those carbs are harmful enough on the metabolic system, but they have an insidious cardiovascular effect as well when combined with all that saturated fat. Heart disease loves the po' boy.

With gut bombs like that being grabbed hand over fist like beads during Mardi Gras, it should surprise no one that diabetes has cut a swath through New Orleans no less devastating than Katrina's. In 2007, the Louisiana Public Health Institute conducted a phone survey to determine just how bad the diabetes problem in the city had become. Nine percent of those eighteen and older reported having been diagnosed with the disease. This number, of course, would only reflect those who *know* they're diabetic. The actual number is surely higher.

For now, anyway, my intellect presides over my lizard brain as I sit down by myself for dinner at La Bayou Restaurant and ask for a glass of cabernet sauvignon, my favorite. I proceed to order a filet mignon, blackened and medium-rare. The entrée comes with steamed vegetables and a baked potato, offered plain or loaded with the works. I'm curious as to what heights of dietary decadence "the works" would reach here in the French Quarter, but those elements don't worry me. What does is the baked potato, so I skip that. The waitress offers to double the amount of vegetables, which seems pointless but not worth the effort of declining. I'll leave the basket of bread on the table untouched.

After I've finished, the waitress asks if I'd like to see the dessert tray. I would, but I won't.

Beyond all the science being presented at the ADA conference, type 2 diabetes really boils down to the sum total of a very long trail of personal choices, made over a lifetime. Whether you worked the treadmill for twenty minutes or turned on the television. Whether you stuck with your diet or ordered that fudge brownie with vanilla ice cream, promising yourself that you would repent later. The truth is, by the time you have or even flirt with type 2 diabetes, there's probably a lot more out of whack in your life than just your blood sugar. That certainly was the case with me.

2

BETWEEN THE DEVIL
AND THE DNA

had been thumbing through a magazine at a newsstand in Westwood, California, when something made me look to my left. Ten feet away, stepping from the street onto the sidewalk with his familiar gait, was my father, dressed in a suit. He had gained a few pounds and lost a lot of hair since I had last seen him. That had been several years earlier.

We were both startled. Embarrassed too, since we hadn't called each other, let alone seen each other, in so very long. I don't remember what we said. I know we exchanged phone numbers, but the reunion was as short-lived as it was random. This was the late 1980s, when I was a graduate student at UCLA. Our next encounter wouldn't occur for another two decades.

I completed my degree and after that was busy carving out a career in publishing. I was hell-bent on forging my own life and oblivious to my father's whereabouts. Uninterested, even. On rare occasions I'd hear a story about him at a family gathering. He had become an entrepreneur. He had made a lot of money. He had lost a lot of money. He had made it back again. He had remarried. He had a new family that included four children, none of whom knew that he had three sons from a prior marriage. Each report triggered only a glint of bewilderment, then indifference. It wasn't simply that I hadn't seen Tom O'Connell in two decades; he had been cast out of my mind.

Until September 2006, that is. My father's brother, my uncle Hughie, was on the phone. He said that my father lay in intensive care in a Los Angeles hospital. Two consecutive operations had removed most of his right leg. Diabetes.

Word of my father's condition saddened and sickened me. But I processed the news the same way I might a shocking Internet headline or TV bulletin—with my brain, not with my heart. This tragic news offered one more piece, perhaps the final piece, of a puzzle whose component parts had never seemed to form a coherent picture, even though I had inherited many of those same pieces.

Not surprisingly, given the traumatic nature of such an operation, my father's life was imperiled. "If you want to see your father again, now's the time," Uncle Hughie said.

But now wasn't the time. Not for me. In fact, the thought of making the trip from Pennsylvania to Los Angeles never entered my mind. It would be another year and a half later, in February 2008, when I'd board a flight to L.A. to see Tom O'Connell. And even then, I told myself I was going on business. I was writing a story about my own blood sugar problems for *Men's Health*, and I believed sharing my own experience could alert unsuspecting readers to the disease that had cost my father his leg. As for him, I had neither received nor wanted one ounce of support since he and my mother divorced during my senior year in high school and I headed off to UCLA. He owed me absolutely nothing, but for the first time—selfishly, perhaps—I wanted something from him: a cautionary tale for my story and the magazine's readers.

My flight touched down in L.A., and I checked into a hotel near LAX before noon. At 2:00 P.M., I was scheduled to reunite with my father at a nursing home in Chatsworth, which lies at the northwest end of the San Fernando Valley. L.A. real estate prices push working-class families to the peripheries of adjacent valleys, and Chatsworth runs the gamut from strip malls and industrial parks to horse properties and single-story ranch homes. You'd never know it from looking at the generic building facades that this community also lays claim to being the Hollywood of the adult-film industry.

I didn't know what twists and turns my father's life had taken over the last two decades, but he hadn't ended up very far from where he was back when I knew him. Twenty minutes north of Chatsworth lay the Santa Clarita Valley, the destination for the last of the ten relocations my father had orchestrated during my childhood. Ten minutes to the south of Chatsworth is Woodland Hills, where I had worked for *Muscle & Fitness* during the late 1990s, early 2000s, and again in 2005.

If my father had been living near Chatsworth all these years, we probably had passed within a few blocks of each other dozens of times during the past decade.

When I entered the hotel room, I slung my duffel bag onto the bed. After ordering lunch from room service, I dialed my father's number. No answer. I tried again twenty minutes later. Ditto. I shot off a text to a friend of mine in New York City. CAN'T BELIEVE IT, it read. I THINK MY FATHER IS STANDING ME UP ONE LAST TIME.

After eating, I dialed the number again. This time, the rings stopped at two. Silence. After a few seconds, a faint voice emerged. It was my father. The two sentences he managed to utter were enough to let me know that we would meet.

Forty-five minutes later, I was guiding my rental car onto the northbound lanes of the San Diego Freeway, better known as the 405. In light of our serial moves as a family, I've often wondered if this city had been pulling my father into its orbit all along. Or maybe when he reached the Pacific Ocean, he simply had no place left to run. Regardless, when my father arrived at what would become his final destination, he unpacked his family and started another.

Like him, I had always found L.A. intoxicating and irresistible. In hindsight, I must have responded to the city's indifference to tradition and encouragement of reinvention. In that sense, I shared my father's wanderlust, albeit with a twist. His changes tended to be geographical; my restlessness took the form of personal transformation.

Since I had traveled this route so many times in the past, cruising north along the 405—past the Getty Museum on the left and then descending into the San Fernando Valley—temporarily put me at ease, even though I didn't know what to expect when I arrived. This shaky, tentative reunion was past the point of no return, however, as I exited the 405, banked onto an overpass, and merged onto the 118 Freeway, westbound. My father and my past were now minutes away. My stomach churned.

After several wrong turns, I pulled up to the curb of the Chatsworth Park Care Center, a white, single-story complex. I walked inside and became lost; I inherited my father's glucose metabolism but my mother's sense of direction. Turning a corner, I spied a nurses' station. I told the woman seated behind the counter that I was here to see Tom O'Connell, that I was his son, and she told me his room number. I strolled down the hall, past patients in wheelchairs staring blankly at TV screens, and arrived at his room. I knew my father would look starkly different—and much, much worse—than I remembered, but the person before me was unrecognizable. Even though he was in a fetal curl and swaddled with blankets, I could tell this man was no more than six feet tall. And his face was rounded, not angular, like my father's. Actually . . . this wasn't my father at all.

I made my way back to the nurses' station and told the woman what had happened. She looked down at her paperwork. "Oh, you mean the other Tom O'Connell," she said. "We have two patients here by that name. The one missing his leg, right?"

The next room I entered was the correct one. I knew this because the first thing I saw was a prosthetic leg propped against a wall. As I passed a curtain, the man I beheld looked nothing like the man who had raised me, and yet it was unmistakably him. Two decades will change anyone, but he showed none of the grace or subtle shadings of aging; this was a human body in the process of cannibalizing itself. I've had little experience with death, but my father looked like what I'd expect a man to look like in his casket.

Then his eyes moved. From his hospital bed, my father struggled to size me up, angling his neck like a man peering hard into a foggy mirror. He had not only lost much of his body weight, but in a particularly cruel twist, he'd even lost a tall man's defining characteristic, his stature. Where his right leg should have been was a brown corduroy pant leg, folded up and pinned together. Formerly six foot three, and 215 pounds, he was now a 145-pound collection of bones jutting against crinkled, discolored flesh.

He smiled, and I was taken aback that this once-handsome man now had rotten teeth and horribly inflamed gums, more evidence of sugar's corrosive power.

My father extended his blood-splotched arm, his firm handshake now a feeble grasp. "It's good to see you, Jeff," he said. "I'm glad you came."

"It's great to see you too, Dad. How ya feelin'?"

I cringed inside at my own question, and his face winced, perhaps the best way he could summarize all he had endured. "It's been kind of rough. But I'm glad you came." He continued to hold my hand, punctuating sentences like that one with a gentle squeeze.

Shifting his weight in bed seemed to require all of his remaining strength, and while he closed his eyes to summon it, I looked around. A small Phillies pennant was tacked above his bed. I saw a few photographs of children, no doubt his children, although they were strangers to me. I noticed a yellow balloon tethered to the bed frame. *Shit, it was his birthday last week.* It was the sort of detail I had long since forgotten.

"Your brother tells me you're a writer, and a successful one. He showed me some of your articles and books."

"Yeah, well, it's a good thing, because I can't do anything else." He smiled.

Twenty years leaves a lot of ground to cover. You have to start somewhere. He wanted to know some basic information. This wasn't the time to ask the questions I wanted answered. Maybe the right time for that would never come.

"Are you married?" he said.

"Nope, not yet, although I've come close once or twice."

When a conversational lull arrived after several minutes, we switched

over instinctively to baseball. Some things never change between a father and son, I guess. Baseball remained our default topic, just as it had
been when I was seven years old.

His alertness surprised me. I wasn't sure if that was good or bad now
that diabetes was running the show. Although it was turned off, a TV
sat on the bureau across from his bed. He must have been following
current events.

"Who are you for in the election?" he asked.

"Obama," I said. I asked him the same question, knowing the answer.

"McCain," he said, about to begin the elaborate process of shifting
once again. "But I can see why people like him," he said, referring to
Obama. It wasn't the innocuous statement that it might seem. I thought
back to conversations overheard as a child when the adults around me
didn't think an African-American was fit to quarterback a football team,
let alone a nation. So many of my father's beliefs—his religion, his poli-
tics, his views on race—weren't ones that I'd adopted myself. That didn't
drive us apart, though.

"So how long have you been diabetic, Dad?" I asked. I knew that
anyone in his current state would be nearing the end of a long and gru-
eling battle with this disease.

He thought. "I don't really know," he said. "I didn't really watch my
blood sugars. I passed out one day. I don't remember anything after that."
His voice trailed off.

"You didn't have symptoms in your forties, fifties, and sixties?"

"No," he said. It felt like the sort of lie I might have told him as a
teenager. I would later learn that he had neglected his diabetes for at
least a decade.

After several more minutes of conversation, all he could muster were
short phrases—"I love you," "It's great to see you"—and he repeated
them several times. So did I. I had no desire to delve any deeper, under
the circumstances. Nor, I suspect, did he. After what he had been through,
what mattered was making him feel as comfortable as possible. The
past and future didn't seem to matter much, given that the here and
now was *this*.

As I was preparing to leave, a pair of orderlies wheeled in a dinner of chicken, mashed potatoes, and fruit juice. They pricked his finger and measured his blood sugar, but the key is what happens *after* a diabetic eats. My father bypassed the chicken and went straight for the potatoes and juice, relishing a moment's pleasure. It wasn't the time or place to say anything—again, whatever brightened his mood had value—but I was taken aback that fast-acting sugars were on the menu for a diabetic.

"When I was working in a hospital, I'd see diabetics receive their insulin, after which their blood sugar would drop," says Keith W. Berkowitz, M.D., medical director of the Center for Balanced Health in New York City. "So they'd be given orange juice, their blood sugar would rise and fall again, they'd get more insulin, then more orange juice—they'd go back and forth all day. That's exactly what you want to avoid—chasing it up and down. Because once you fall behind at breakfast, you're never going to catch up." From diabetes' onset until a patient's death, the medical community takes a backward dietary approach to this dietary disease, with deadly results.

In addition to the dubious carbohydrate-laden meals served to him at his care facility, my father pointed out his root beer stash in a cabinet across the room. He still indulged this diabetic's poison even knowing that too much sugar cost him a limb. This scene reminded me of a drug addict who has seen his life destroyed by the substance he can't refuse. Only the worse off he becomes, the lousier he feels, the more he craves the very thing that sentenced him to this hell on earth.

DIABETES WOULD HAVE been the last fate you would have predicted for my father if you had met him when he was a teenager. The year was 1952, and New Jersey had its own version of the story told in the movie *Hoosiers*. That film was set in 1954, but two years before that, my father became his own team's Jimmy Chitwood, the fictionalized character who didn't suit up until his senior year but led his team to the state title.

My father's true passion was baseball, not basketball. That helps to explain why he, like Jimmy Chitwood, didn't play for his high school basketball team until his senior year, and only after a coach in dire need of a center saw him scoring at will in gym class. "I used to horse around with a basketball in gym class, but I didn't like the structure of practices and drills," my father told me. "I'd score sixty points or so in these playground games, so one day the coach strode up to me and said: 'We need a center. Be at practice on Monday morning.' It wasn't a request; it was an order."

My father was an unlikely giant killer. In photographs from his high school yearbook, Tom O'Connell's tousled mop of hair, recoiling body language, and disaffected expression appear better suited for a leather jacket and dangling cigarette than a basketball uniform. Even in the 1950s, a six-foot-three pivot man was undersized, but he stood tallest on a team of runts representing Merchantville High School, the namesake of a small town nestled along the Jersey side of the Schuylkill, across from Philadelphia. Personality-wise, my father was a study in highs and lows: He could be moody and withdrawn, but once he stepped onto the court, Tucker, as he was known, became a crazy firebrand, the kind of player who would slam his elbow into a taller defender's rib cage if that stood between him and the rim. In short, he was exactly the sort of human incendiary device capable of igniting a band of underdogs on a Cinderella run. This temperament would serve him less well later in life, however.

After an unremarkable regular season, Merchantville slipped into New Jersey's state basketball tournament with little fanfare and even less of a chance to win even a game or two. Once the tournament began, however, they caught fire, knocking off larger foes such as Camden High and Woodrow Wilson one after the other behind my father's deadly left-handed hook shot and the pesky guard tandem of Ray La Greca and Little Ed Brown. "The squad overturned many big apple carts," as the high school yearbook writer would put it. The team wound up winning the South Jersey Championship.

From there, it was on to the New Jersey State Championships. The ending to this storybook season was bittersweet, with Merchantville losing its final game. The difference between victory and defeat turned on one errant bounce and a single point.

After high school, Tom O'Connell joined the army as a military policeman. All he really guarded were opposing players as a member of a barnstorming military squad stocked mostly with former collegiates from schools such as Vanderbilt and Kentucky. After my father's tour of duty ended, a military contact arranged a tryout for him with Marshall University in West Virginia. The school was set to hand my father a scholarship until officials reviewed his high school transcript. Apparently he didn't like the structure of the classroom, either. He was asked to spend a semester at a nearby junior college trying to improve his grades, but he became homesick and left, a decision he would regret.

Basketball was over, but life was about to tip off.

As a player, my father thrived under the wing of a skilled high school basketball coach, a man by the name of Bob Elder. His real fathers offered no such constructive coaching, however. When my father was eighteen months old, his biological father, Thomas Joseph O'Connell Sr., left his wife pregnant with twins. Five years later, he was drafted to fight in World War II and disappeared for forty years, the beginning of a family tradition. The stepfather who entered my father's life at age seven resented supporting another man's three children and ruled his new roost with crushing authority, unleashing beatings with thick horse reins, a souvenir brought home from soldiering in Germany.

The childhood memories I hold of my father are much better, except for his occasionally hair-trigger temper and the butt whippings it could produce; and his wanderlust, which made me the new kid at school seemingly every year. My father did fatherly things, such as playing sports with my two brothers and me, often and well. He coached our basketball teams. If the cancer my father beat when he was thirty-seven and I was nine had taken his life instead, to this day, my memories of him would have been affectionate, loving, and idealized: *This was the best dad.*

At moments, in his own way, he was.

NOW, THIS. I can't possibly understand how my father must have felt lying in that bed in such a state. I've never endured a single moment even approaching the misery he was now experiencing every waking second. But I knew how he felt at the earlier stages of the disease, despite his denial of having ever had symptoms—the sort of denial that landed him at the mercy of a surgeon's saw.

Fifteen months earlier, and a week or so after receiving the call about my father's amputation, I was attending a previously scheduled doctor's appointment, a follow-up to a physical exam. I had sought an assessment of my health. I was wondering if there was some way to make my body function a little better, some antidote to disparate symptoms that made me feel sluggish, particularly in the mornings, and particularly after I had had a pizza or a burger and fries for dinner the night before.

Like many men, I had simply asked a colleague—in my case, one of the editors of *Men's Health*—for a recommendation. I made this crucial health decision with as much deliberation as one would give to choosing a garage for an oil change. The editor directed me to Sam Bub & Associates, a folksy small-town practice whose clientele included a number of the magazine's staff members. When I entered the clinic for the first time, I met with Todd H., M.D., a rotund man with thinning hair and a penchant for bad jokes told at awkward moments, like during medical exams. A clipboard and stethoscope weren't the only baggage Dr. H. carried into the examination room. An extra fifty pounds or so settled around his waist.

As part of our initial visit, he had the nurse draw some blood for routine lab work. Like all patients, I was weighed as a matter of course, and my height was measured for the umpteenth time. It hasn't changed since I reached six feet, six inches as a twenty-one-year-old. Height and weight allow for the calculation of a person's body mass index (BMI), a number that's supposed to tell if you're overweight. Unfortunately, BMI doesn't account for body composition, the ratio between muscle and fat mass. An individual standing five foot ten might work out every day but weigh the same as someone of similar stature who sits around all day. The difference: one is accumulating muscle, while the other is hoarding fat. Even though they might have a matching BMI, it is misleading to lump together such disparate populations.

Fresh on the heels of hearing about my father, I had returned to

Dr. H.'s office for the results. After some introductory banter, he opened a file folder and began scanning the results. Then he looked up.

"Does diabetes run in your family?" he asked.

It doesn't take more than a split second to fill in the blanks when a doctor poses a leading question about a disease, especially when you're skinny and the doctor is asking about type 2 diabetes, which is normally associated with the overweight.

This wasn't idle chatter.

I had scored 116 milligrams per deciliter (mg/dL) on my fasting plasma glucose test, indicative of prediabetes. Ten points higher, and I'd do away with the *pre*.

Not to say that this bad medical news came as a huge surprise. Both of my parents had survived cancer. My mother has had epileptic seizures as well. But I was tall and lean. Guys used to kid that I'd need to run around in the shower just to get wet. Diabetes? As life-threatening diseases go, leprosy and typhoid fever ranked higher on my things-that-might-kill-me list, even in light of the news I had learned about my father only a week earlier.

I'll be damned. How the hell could I have missed the signs?

I left the doctor's office in a fog. I looked at my legs as I walked back to my car. Would I, too, lose one of them eventually? After sliding behind the wheel, I sat still for a moment and closed my eyes, trying to imagine the claustrophobia of a darkness that would never lift. Would impotence lie somewhere in my future as well? Adding up everything that diabetes could take away sobered me. I realized that in the end this disease could leave a man with nothing but regret.

That grim thought must loop through my father's mind dozens, if not hundreds, of times a day, I thought. *Then again, maybe he doesn't think of it at all*. During the drive back through Emmaus to the *Men's Health* offices, my thoughts were filled with my past, not my muddled present, or even a future that had just turned overcast. Like many skinny people whose blood sugar regulation goes haywire, I had misinterpreted being thin for being healthy. I had a hunch that my DNA wasn't centenarian material—men in my extended family are often buried too early—but I didn't think I was booby-trapping my own body. I had never smoked.

Recreational drugs and excessive drinking held no interest for me. I wasn't overweight. My lifestyle seemed comparatively healthy to me, a fact I thought would help stack the odds against premature sickness and disease. Yet over those two decades, I had somehow acquired a disease of the overweight, or at least what I *thought* was a disease only for the overweight. Unfortunately I had been eating a lot of unhealthy foods with impunity because they didn't cause me to pack on pounds. But they were unhealthy nonetheless.

It wasn't until I collaborated with a dietitian on her nutrition book for men, *Power Food*, published in 2004, that I began squaring away my diet. I knew enough to realize that aging alone would make my body less forgiving of careless eating. So I traded in some of the fast food I had relied on for years for healthier foods, or at least what I had always been told were healthy: yogurt, milk, Gatorade, pasta, wheat bread, and the like. Yet even those supposed upgrades, as it turns out, were roiling my blood sugar. After working out at the gym, I'd swing by 7-Eleven for a Butterfinger or an Almond Joy and a twenty-ounce bottle of Gatorade, the popular workout drink. The first combination contains 78 grams of carbs, 64 of them in the form of sugars. For the second combination—an Almond Joy and a Gatorade—the numbers are 61 and 55, respectively. Unleashing those simple sugars in my bloodstream right before bed was wreaking havoc on my metabolic system.

For all I know, diabetes was announcing its intention to strike me back when I was a pockmarked, cavity-riddled teen. In a study published in the *American Journal of Clinical Nutrition*, researchers divided a group of young pimpletons into two groups. The control was fed a diet heavy in processed carbs, what they probably favored before the study. The other group was not allowed to eat white bread and other refined carbs; instead they relied on a hunter-gatherer's diet of lean meat, fish, fruits, vegetables, and low-fat dairy. The latter group proved far more likely to see their blemishes vanish. The experiment reverse-engineered an anthropological observation—the absence of acne in traditional hunting societies, from South America to Australia and the Pacific Islands. That is, until they switch menus. "Once you place them on a Western diet that's high in easily digestible carbohydrates, which are not part of the traditional hunter's diet, acne appears," says Neil J. Mann, Ph.D., nutrition professor at RMIT University in Melbourne, Australia. "So it's not genetic; it's something their prior diet protected them from."

Mann believes your mother was right when she nagged about sugar causing a skin breakout. Insulin and the other growth factors produced in response to carbs affect hormones in the skin, thickening pores. Once the pores seal off, they fill with oil and become infected.

I also thought back to high school, when my slender body didn't seem efficient at producing energy for basketball practices or games. During "suicide" drills or distance slogs through the hundred-plus low-desert heat north of Los Angeles, the guards and forwards would pass me on their way back. In hindsight, my metabolic system might have been burning through glucose so fast that my body could never store much of it for later use. I could tell I wasn't built for endurance.

Even hair loss, which I've held in check with prescription and over-the-counter meds since my college years, may be a harbinger of insulin resistance rather than just a pain in the neck. Researchers at the Institute of Endocrinology in Prague analyzed the blood glucose levels of thirty men with hair loss predating their thirtieth birthday. Those guys were more likely to be in the early stages of diabetes than men with thick hair. The researchers speculated that male-pattern baldness could be the male equivalent of polycystic ovary syndrome (PCOS) in women, with insulin resistance as the root cause of both. A bigger study of 740 men between the ages of forty and ninety-one—conducted by a pair of Taiwanese researchers and published online in spring 2010—found a significant association between hair loss and the metabolic abnormalities that are synonymous with insulin resistance. Other studies have found similar links.

Warning signs had been flashing before I visited Dr. H., but I didn't connect them with one another or to type 2 diabetes. I thought it was stress. In 2005 I had been promoted twice within four months to become the editor in chief of *Muscle & Fitness* magazine, and had left behind my then girlfriend to move from Jersey City to Southern California. I hadn't had a day of management experience, and the staff of griping underachievers I inherited from my predecessor didn't help matters. From the middle of the summer into fall and winter, stress was my shadow.

One weekend morning in November, I woke up and drank a glass of water . . . and then another . . . and then another. I felt as if I had consumed gallons before the weekend was out. Still, my thirst couldn't be quenched. I knew this wasn't normal, yet I didn't think about diabetes, even though thirst is a classic clue, one people should know to connect with diabetes. I would score a prediabetic 116 mg/dL on the fasting plasma glucose test nine months later, but I suspect I had already passed the line demarcating diabetes, 126 mg/dL, more than a few times before, including that weekend. In fact nearly a quarter century may have elapsed between the beginning of my insulin resistance and my prediabetes diagnosis. How much damage had occurred during that time, I didn't know.

While the link between blood sugar ills and stress is harder to quantify than more easily measured triggers such as sugar or sloth, a link does exist. In stressful situations, your body releases another hormone, cortisol. Hormones deliver messages, and this one warns your body of trouble ahead. The secretion of cortisol sets off a chain reaction prompting the liver to ready glucose as fuel, and releasing fat energy for use by muscles. Your body is ensuring that your brain and central nervous system have enough energy to handle whatever problem might arise.

Just as consumed sugar needs shuttling into cells, so too does the glucose released by the liver in response to cortisol. For the insulin resistant, that glucose will be equally hard to handle.

You don't have to be a deadline-crunched magazine editor to be stressed-out enough to disrupt your glucose metabolism, sending your blood sugar on a roller-coaster ride. The world's a complicated place; stress is everywhere. Some of it's necessary—otherwise, we wouldn't be able to function—but too much can harm the body. People often don't realize this until their body breaks down.

Runaway stress, unquenchable thirst—my body was *already* beginning to break down. Which is why getting fired from *Muscle & Fitness*
in late 2005 may have saved my life.

I TOOK A few months to coauthor another book and then scored a job
at *Men's Health*. It was May 2006 and time for my second cross-country
move in a year. I went online to Google Maps, entered "from" Woodland Hills, California, "to" Zionsville, Pennsylvania, hit a button on my
keyboard, and grabbed the printout as I hurried out to my car. (Planning has never been my strongest suit.) I was starting my new job in
four days, so all I needed was the quickest way from point A to B. Each
morning would dawn with no specific stopping point en route to my
final destination. I'd drive all day and push into the night until fatigue
made continuing impossible.

While my diet had improved, thanks to information I picked up as a
fitness writer, trips such as this were tailor-made for backsliding to the
dietary indiscretions of my youth. Driving fifteen hours a day meant ordering meals from drive-through speakers. A typical fast-food meal for
me was a Big Mac with a large order of french fries, washed down with
a large Coca-Cola Classic. The fallout from this gut bomb: 1,350 calories and 194 grams of carbs, including 95 grams of sugar. I'd hit the
Arby's drive-through and grab a large roast beef sandwich and a large
chocolate shake, totaling 1,058 calories and 151 grams of carbohydrates,
112 grams of which were sugar. Not to mention all the saturated fat and
sodium in those meals.

Even those carb loads pale, though, next to the premium fish fillet
sandwich, large original chocolate Frosty, and medium french fries I
purchased one evening at Wendy's. The stat sheet for this diet disaster
tallied 1,840 calories, 78 grams of fat (18 of it saturated, 1.5 of it trans),
80 grams of cholesterol, 2,660 milligrams of sodium, 236 grams of
carbs, 8 grams of dietary fiber, 79 grams of sugar, and 51 grams of protein. That meal should come with an arterial stent rather than a straw.

I'd scarf down one of these meals, or something equally unhealthful,
and be back on the road without ever having unbuckled my seat belt.

I might as well have shot up with some drug before guiding my car back onto the highway, so powerful are the effects exerted by that many carbs on a body like mine. Fatigue didn't set in gradually; it hit me with a *whoosh*, as if I had popped a Vicodin or been shot with a tranquilizer capable of felling a large predator. Before I knew it, my nerves felt like they were shutting down. I'd wait for the first cluster of hotel signs glowing near a freeway off-ramp, check into a room, and free-fall onto the bed, often still in my street clothes. Some nights I swear I was sound asleep the instant my head hit the pillow.

The day before I was to start work, I rolled across the Pennsylvania Turnpike and its carpets of green forest, a lovely flashback to my youth. Late in the afternoon, armed with directions and a garage door code, I wound my way back through farm country en route to Zionsville, a small town located a few miles southwest of Allentown. Founded in 1762 as a rural village of the Pennsylvania Dutch, Allentown became a bustling population center during the Industrial Revolution, based on iron production for railroads. Booms and busts have taken turns ever since. The railroad bubble popped in 1873, but by the 1900s, Allentown's economy had found new footing, with companies churning out everything from silk and parlor furniture to beer and cigars. In the postwar era, the economy sagged again as manufacturing headed offshore. Currently officials are trying to revitalize the city by attracting new business into the downtown district, an effort that doesn't appear to be taking hold.

Around a bend, a beautiful white house loomed to my right. I pulled into the driveway of the Powder Valley Mill, a four-story house whose shingle roof angled up to a crow's nest. To the left stood a red barn. A stone's throw beyond it was a small body of water.

After parking my car in the driveway, I ventured onto the deck behind the house. Before me lay the mill's secret: a forested ravine bisected by a stream meandering around rocks and boulders. To my right, the stream disappeared into a stone tunnel, above which ran railroad tracks that curved off into the forest. To my left was the stream's source: a thirty-foot-high waterfall flowing over a stone dam that bounded a large pond—the water I had spied past the barn. A moss-covered wooden bridge crossed the stream fifty feet from the waterfall. If this place marked the transition from my past life to my future, I was eager to find out what lay on the other side.

Despite this postcardlike setting, my first spring and summer in eastern Pennsylvania felt stressful and uncertain. In L.A. I had reached the pinnacle of the muscle-magazine business, for whatever that's worth, but making the transition to a mainstream magazine such as *Men's Health* felt like a promotion from Double-A ball to the major leagues. I was only the second executive writer in the magazine's twenty-year history, a span when it had become the most successful men's title in the country. After several months, I still wasn't sure that I had what it would take to succeed in this position.

My new job wasn't my only concern. My body felt as if it had been unplugged from a wall socket. Rising from bed became a frustrating struggle. Before I had even lifted my head from the pillow, a band of pain would clamp around my skull. This early-morning sluggishness often made me late for work. Headaches dogged me to where I was popping Extra-Strength Tylenol capsules like popcorn. My joints were achy and sore, particularly around where my left leg joined my hip. The pain could stab so sharply that I'd have to give the leg a little tug to begin exiting my car.

With diabetes no outward deformity, no internal alarm bells, announce that something is definitely wrong. At first the symptoms don't even feel like symptoms, they're so mundane, general, and vague. This hurts. That aches. Something feels weird, but what is it, exactly? And even when the symptoms become harder to dismiss, they can still be dismissed as the price paid for a stressed-out, overworked life or simply aging. U.K. researchers have found that eating a carb-packed meal may cause people with poor glucose tolerance to become grouchier and more forgetful, a finding to which I can personally attest. But good luck separating the effects of a single meal from the twenty other things that make so many of us feel out of sorts in the morning.

Only with hindsight did the severe headaches, fatigue, and bouts of unquenchable thirst become recognizable as diabetes-on-the-march. What I hadn't done yet was connect any of the dots in a way that would have alerted me to the danger lurking.

To his credit, Dr. H. made a correct diagnosis of this health threat based on my blood work. I was prediabetic, and he told me that. A sense of both dread and relief comes with learning the true nature of what's really going on inside your body. Now I finally knew why my body was feeling the way that it did.

But a diagnosis is not a cure.

3

WHITE COATS, WHITE FLAGS

Perhaps because I've confronted the disease myself, I've come to view type 2 diabetes as a tap on the shoulder, one that presents an amazing opportunity for any individual to turn around his or her life. But there's a larger, societal picture, and it's not pretty. The number of people in the United States with diabetes has reached 26.8 million, according to 2009 data estimates released by the IDF. The number with prediabetes is more than twice that. Diabetes is increasing at an alarming rate among men and women of all ages.

So when does a doctor tell a patient that he or she has type 2 diabetes? Because the disease is chronic, progressive, and stealthy, a diagnosis is not always a yes-or-no proposition, as it is with many ailments. Blood sugar readings fall along a continuum, and the cutoff points for type 2 diabetes have periodically been changed, as strange as that sounds. The trend has been for these cutoff points to be lowered, which, of course, multiplies the ranks overnight. Over time, diabetes researchers have found that even slight elevations in blood glucose harm the body. Hence the disease has to be redefined.

Regardless of where the cutoff points for diabetes fall at a given time, large populations can't be divided between diabetics and nondiabetics based on a single number. That's because no single number triggers diabetic complications in every individual. One person with a fasting plasma glucose score of 120 mg/dL might feel asymptomatic, although damage likely would be under way. Another person at 120 might just feel kind of blah and out of sorts. A third person with that score might be really thirsty and peeing more than normal, both classic diabetes symptoms. When blood sugar builds up in the bloodstream, the body wants to get rid of it, stat. So it sends you to the bathroom, for repeated trips if necessary.

Do any of these individuals have type 2 diabetes? Based on that one blood test score, all, some, or none of them might. At a minimum, they're all at least prediabetic, a sugarcoated term for the fifty-seven million people in the United States whose blood sugar is creeping toward diabetes but not over the line. However, the odds are sky high that someone with prediabetes will lose the prefix within ten years, probably sooner rather than later.

Blood glucose should be at its lowest after fasting, so elevation on this test spells trouble. A score of 100 to 125 mg/dL equals prediabetes, assuming a follow-up test confirms the first one—which holds true for most diagnostic tests for diabetes, so I won't mention that qualifier again. Above that range is diabetes; score below 100 and at or above 70, and the doctor probably will say that your blood sugar is "normal," meaning healthy. But it might not be healthy at all.

Type 2 diabetes can be diagnosed in other ways. If you had a finger prick, a test strip, and a glucose meter, you could set this book down and test your blood glucose right now. That would be called a random (as opposed to fasting) plasma glucose test. ER doctors testing your blood sugar on the spot would be another random test. No allowance is made for whether you last ate three hours ago or had pasta for lunch ten minutes ago. On a random glucose test, a score of 200 mg/dL or higher indicates diabetes, especially if accompanied by symptoms such as increased thirst, excessive urination, and blurred vision.

Both of these tests provide some information, and that beats ignorance. Yet they're more limited than many doctors are willing to admit or even realize. Blood glucose levels fluctuate in response to nutritional status, activity level, stress, and other factors, even as you sleep. The climbs and descents can be steep and rapid. The random and fasting tests offer only one reading taken at one moment in time. Imagine trying to describe a football play based on one snapshot taken at the line of scrimmage—before the ball is even snapped. That's the level of information here. As a result, you and your doctor may lack a complete picture of what's unfolding inside your body.

This helps to explain how a quarter of U.S. diabetics could remain ignorant of their disease. What you want are leading indicators; in contrast, these standard tests reveal later manifestations of a disease that takes its sweet time in showing itself, while undermining your health. Seven years typically elapse between the onset of type 2 diabetes and its diagnosis, and insulin resistance, the underlying cause, can begin a dozen years before a diabetes diagnosis. So much for early detection.

Perhaps in recognition of this reality, the ADA decided in late 2009 to approve a test called A1C—which had been designed to monitor glucose control—for diagnostic purposes as well. This test measures how much glucose attaches itself to a certain protein in red blood cells. The amount is expressed as a percentage. A1C levels between 5.7 percent and 6.4 percent are considered prediabetes; anything higher is full-on diabetes. Since red blood cells stay in the body for two to three months, A1C represents an average over time. Diabetes experts often present this test as being close to foolproof, but it's anything but, as I would learn firsthand.

A final way of diagnosing type 2 diabetes and prediabetes is by drinking a sugary solution as the trigger for a metabolic "stress test," or glucose tolerance test. Someone whose blood sugar shoots to 200 mg/dL or above two hours after ingesting the drink is said to have diabetes. If the two-hour score is 140 to 199, the person is said to have "impaired glucose tolerance," which is a fancier way of saying prediabetes.

A glucose tolerance test finally gives some indication of how that hypothetical football play unfolds. Drinking the sugar is like the snapping of the ball. This test also quantifies insulin levels to go along with blood glucose measures, revealing the interaction between the two. That brochure from Sanofi-Aventis says that "insulin is only a part of treating diabetes"; what it doesn't say is that too much insulin is a big part of the problem, whether it's coming from an injection or your own pancreas. Everyone knows high blood sugar is a bad actor in diabetes, but another killer is excessive internal insulin production, which can corrode the inside of arteries, feed tumors, and set the stage for rheumatoid arthritis, among a whole host of ills.

Which makes me wonder: Why on Earth would you want to be shooting more of the stuff into your body if you didn't absolutely have to?

WHAT'S ASTOUNDING IS that when you combine the numbers for type 2 diabetes and its precursor, prediabetes, one in three adults in the United States now has a blood sugar abnormality that places them on the path for truly horrific diabetes-related complications. One in three! Ominously, type 2 diabetes is also setting its sights on the young in record numbers. A study in *Diabetes Care* found that between 1993 and 2004, hospital stays for diabetes among those twenty-nine years or younger increased nearly 40 percent. Eventually those stays will be for heart and kidney transplants. At the current pace, one in every three people born in the United States in the year 2000 will become diabetic. For minorities, the rate will be one in two.

Aside from the toll in human misery, the cost of diabetes is threatening our health care system with collapse, which will have dire consequences for our broader economy and financial system. The U.S. diabetes tab for only direct medical expenditures comes to nearly $120 billion a year. Throw in lost productivity—$58 billion worth of missed workdays, lackluster job performance, and the lost input of those who can't work at all any longer—and the total price tag rises to nearly $178 billion. Government programs are very hard hit: Obesity and diabetes now devour more than 30 percent of Medicare's budget, a number that would be much higher if all the cardiovascular disease caused by insulin resistance were properly attributed.

We have plenty of company too; our national epidemic is really a global pandemic. Type 2 diabetes affects 285 million people worldwide, according to the IDF, and their estimate may well fall on the low side, since the disease is so hard to detect. One person around the world develops diabetes every five seconds, swelling the ranks by more than seventeen thousand a day. That's more than seven million new cases of diabetes a year. The World Health Organization expects the number of people with diabetes worldwide to double by 2030. Distant lands are gaining ground on the United States economically, but many of them are acquiring our morbidities at an even faster pace.

One reason is that for the first time in human history, the overweight outnumber the malnourished. "Diabetes, along with obesity, is looming as the biggest epidemic in human history," says Paul Zimmet, M.D., Ph.D., director of international research at the Baker IDI Heart and Diabetes Institute in Australia.

Food technology moves much faster than human evolution; most of our foods are recent inventions, and it takes us humans many, many generations to adjust to shifts in the food supply. If you had to forage for your sugar, like our distant ancestors did, you would have an awfully hard time finding and eating enough fruits, vegetables, and grains to develop type 2 diabetes, especially considering all the energy that the search would take. However, turning in to the drive-through lane of a fast-food establishment demands virtually no energy expenditure; and yet a nearly limitless supply of sugar—buns, fries, sodas, and desserts—instantly comes within reach. Processing allows for huge quantities of sugar and other unhealthy nutrients to hit our system unencumbered by the fiber and other constituents that once made us feel full. As a result, our body's ancient sensors for hunger and satiety are now easily tricked by food technology.

My body certainly fell for it. For too many years, I asked my metabolic system, my body's carburetor, to handle fuel it was never designed to handle.

Eventually, it broke.

The diagnosis of a chronic disease such as type 2 diabetes demands a course of action. So what was my doctor's strategy for ensuring that I would not only reach old age but also navigate it without the assistance of prosthetic limbs and a dialysis regimen? Near the end of our appointment, Dr. H., having told me that I was prediabetic, mumbled something about switching from white rice to brown. He also instructed me to come back in six months for another round of blood work. *Wow, that's it?* I thought. I didn't know much about disease, but managing it seemed like it should require more than tweaking my order at the local Chinese restaurant.

All that I received was a diagnosis, dietary advice so vague and limited as to be woefully inadequate, and the implied sympathy that comes with having a condition that we're taught to believe is destiny for those unfortunate enough to be afflicted. This is consistent with how doctors typically respond to a patient who shows signs of hyperglycemia, which is the technical term for elevated blood glucose levels. "You'll want to watch your blood sugar," they'll say. "It's a little high."

What I didn't receive, and what most patients don't receive, is any advice that would address, let alone fix, the problem, even though dozens of steps can be undertaken to slow or even reverse type 2 diabetes. Unfortunately no one has compiled these steps into an instruction manual for defeating the disease.

The guardian of my wellness didn't ask me what I ate for breakfast, lunch, and dinner every day; nor did he ask how active I was, perhaps assuming that a thin person is by definition physically fit. Unfortunately this missing line of inquiry seems to be the norm, rather than the exception, in doctors' offices. The omission reminded me of something I had learned while researching a feature article on suicide, how mental-health professionals often forget to ask patients and their families the most important question of all: "Is there a gun in your house?"

"It should be medical malpractice for physicians not to ask about lifestyle issues in those situations," says the University of South Carolina's Blair, the man credited with coining the phrase "fat and fit." "Doctors need to know their diabetic patient's activity level. Those diabetics who are obese, but who are at least moderately fit, have a much lower death rate than diabetic patients who are normal weight but unfit." Physical fitness also does a better job than physique shape at predicting who will become a type 2 diabetic in the first place.

The notion that a person can be of normal weight or even skinny but also unfit contradicts society's view of body size and wellness. Yet it's true. One reason is something called visceral fat, the kind that settles around organs rather than spilling over the gut or flapping from the extremities. But excessive visceral fat is also unhealthy. And regardless of their visceral fat levels, a thin person who can't do more than a few minutes on the treadmill is anything but fit. Conversely a study published in *Archives of Internal Medicine* found that half of overweight subjects and one-third of obese subjects were metabolically healthy, lacking many of the major risk factors for heart disease. Another group of researchers writing in the same issue referred to it as "metabolically benign obesity," meaning weight gain divorced from insulin resistance.

At a minimum, doctors should inquire about a patient's physical activity, as Blair urges. That's better than nothing. But just as doctors order lab work that will measure, say, cholesterol levels, they should measure "fitness," which indicates the body's efficiency at taking in and using oxygen. That ability reflects the sum total of a person's habitual physical activity. You and I, as patients, can forget or exaggerate how active we've been of late; a fitness test doesn't lie.

This isn't about submitting to an expensive stress test of the cardio-vascular system. A fitness test can and should be easily accomplished using a cycle ergometer, an apparatus that reveals the working capacity of your heart and lungs. Any YMCA can perform this test; it's no less convenient than going to a lab for blood work. Take the fitness test, and if you don't exercise, the results will speak for themselves.

So fitness gives us a yardstick that's a far, far more important predictor of mortality from diabetes than either body weight or obesity. Yet this measurement is seldom taken. The only beneficiary of this oversight is the disease.

. . .

I LEARNED LITTLE of value about treating this health threat during my initial visit with a seasoned physician. The same sort of sketchy advice that I received is being dispensed to frightened, bewildered diabetics in the offices of doctors across the land. Primary care physicians equate being diabetic with being overweight. Their usual advice is for the patient to unload excess baggage. Unfortunately, thwarting type 2 diabetes involves more than ditching a suitcase, like some gorilla heaving a Samsonite onto the roadside. What's more, most of the diabetes advice doctors offer patients won't rid them of the suitcase even if they are overweight. Losing weight requires specific dietary and exercise techniques, best used in concert, and many doctors don't know what those are, let alone how to implement them.

Prediabetes is a pivot point, the moment when the downward spiral into a life that ends like scenes from a horror movie can still be avoided or at least slowed. But too often, doctors address type 2 diabetes only once it has arrived and advanced, at which point the battle becomes uphill. "Physicians don't know much about prevention," says Michael F. Jacobson, Ph.D., executive director of the Center for Science in the Public Interest in Washington, D.C. "They're taught how to do surgery or which pharmaceuticals are most effective for a particular ailment."

As odd as it sounds, prediabetics like me are more likely to receive useful therapeutic information from a qualified fitness trainer than from a doctor offering no actionable lifestyle advice. Never mind that many trainers know next to nothing about blood sugar themselves; it's just that their healthy-living mantras coincide with the most effective ways to treat prediabetes before its grip becomes a stranglehold.

Many family physicians aren't on the lookout for diabetes's subtle creep, in part because of the limited instruction in the disease they received in medical school. A study published in the official ADA journal *Diabetes Care* found that the curricula of many fourth-year med students fall short of clinical recommendations. That wasn't much of a problem when students were given a patient and told, "Mr. Smith here has type 2 diabetes, so keep an eye on his blood sugar." They knew what to do in that case. The problems arose when Mr. Smith had elevated blood glucose levels but no diagnosis of diabetes. With no label to alert them, the students often missed even severe hyperglycemia.

Medical students still lack sufficient awareness about abnormal blood sugar as full-fledged doctors. One study found that when diabetic patients are discharged from hospitals for a health issue unrelated to blood sugar, their diabetes has been missed at least half the time, in part because half of all diabetics aren't identified as having the disease when admitted. Another study determined that when patients were admitted to a hospital with high blood sugar—but again with no existing diagnosis of diabetes—their chart failed to mention either hyperglycemia or diabetes two-thirds of the time. Diabetes is stealthy, but doctors are supposed to be the detectives who can finger it.

Yet some of them seem clueless when it comes to diagnosing this disease, let alone treating it. One thing I learned early on is that stabbing a vein for blood (a "venous" draw; let the nurse do that) tends to produce a lower blood glucose reading than a finger prick (a "capillary" draw; you can do that at home). The difference can be up to 10 mg/dL, which is significant, considering that the entire range for prediabetes spans only 25 mg/dL. A study published in *Clinical Chemistry* asked doctors how they would interpret a single blood glucose measurement for diagnosis of diabetes. "Many of the doctors didn't understand how to differentiate capillary from venous glucoses, even though diabetes guidelines worldwide clearly mention that these are very different," says Andrea Rita Horvath, M.D., Ph.D., professor of clinical chemistry at University of Szeged in Hungary. "There are several issues we need to teach clinicians when it comes to diagnosing diabetes, and there is a lot of misdiagnosis for that reason."

The limited time doctors spend with patients in the age of managed care also plays right into the disease's hands. "If you spend ten minutes with a patient, how are you going to fix anything?" asks Dr. Berkowitz. "You can barely say hello in that time."

This critique is well worn by now, but diabetes care is a complex subject to teach—and education underpins any effective treatment. "When doctors go in to see diabetics, they might as well have three people sitting in the chair in front of them," says Donald M. Barnett, M.D., who was a staff physician at the Joslin Diabetes Clinic for thirty-five years and is writing a biography of the clinic's namesake. "Diabetes patients are like Siamese triplets." Diabetes is a metabolic disease, an endocrine disease, and a vascular disease all bundled into one. That's just for starters.

Nonetheless many doctors utter a few words of advice and offer a pat on the back, like mine did. In and out prediabetic and diabetic patients go; someone else can deal with the fallout ten years down the road. "Keeping a person from falling off the wagon is hard," says Jacobson. "It takes an ongoing effort, and physicians aren't always the best people to do that. It needs to be a team of exercise physiologists and nurses and dietitians and other specialists. But most communities don't have a system in place to help people adhere to a diet-and-exercise program."

"Centering care on an in-person visit doesn't necessarily help doctors provide good preventive services such as counseling around physical activity," says Randall S. Stafford, M.D., Ph.D., associate professor of medicine at the Stanford Prevention Research Center. "It might be better to have a system where nurses are calling the patient every week, rather than having the patient come in for a fifteen-to-twenty-minute visit with a physician every three months."

That makes sense in light of the major diabetes prevention trials of the past quarter century—such as the aforementioned Diabetes Prevention Program as well as China's Da Qing Diabetes Prevention Study, the Finnish Diabetes Prevention Study, and Look Ahead (Action for Health in Diabetes), a U.S. study. They all tend to confirm one another in finding that those with impaired glucose tolerance are much, much less likely to become diabetic if entered into a lifestyle intervention program of diet, exercise, or both. The default approach is always to make the intervening diet low in fat—that's been the dogma for decades—and I suspect the results would be even more impressive if the diets were made low in carbohydrates. But whenever subjects on the verge of diabetes start exercising, monitoring what they eat, or both, all under supervision, their glucose metabolism will tend to improve.

Another recurring theme in these studies is that the more intensive the intervention, the better the results. That is, patients who interact with study counselors every, say, two weeks do better than those who interact every, say, two months. In the Finnish study, the control group was actually given some basic advice on diet and exercise at the start of the study but little help beyond that. Members of the intervention group received seven individualized nutritional counseling sessions during the first year. On top of those came voluntary group sessions, lectures, cooking lessons, and phone calls checking on their progress in between those seven one-on-one meetings. Subjects could also avail themselves of supervised circuit-training sessions free of charge. The risk of diabetes was reduced by 58 percent in the intensive lifestyle group versus the control group. Someone diagnosed with impaired glucose tolerance or prediabetes usually doesn't even receive that passive advice on diet and exercise that the control group received. So the odds are really stacked against them from the start.

I'm guessing you aren't enrolled in a multicenter randomized clinical trial for a diabetes treatment. But you can apply the same concept to your own life. If you can afford it, see a personal trainer once a week, or a nutritionist once a month. Join a diabetes support group. Can't find one? Start one. I rewarded myself for my diligence at hitting the gym by beginning once-a-week sessions with a lifting coach. I'm pretty fluent in the gym from having worked at *Muscle & Fitness*, but I felt like I needed help to improve my squatting and deadlifting, perhaps because I'm so tall. Those sessions ended up transforming my entire weekly regimen. With exercise, the unintended consequences are almost always positive, and the multiplier effects can transform your life.

I witnessed the benefits of teamwork and interaction while visiting the Joslin Diabetes Center in Boston. Adjacent to Beth Israel Deaconess Medical Center, and affiliated with Harvard Medical Center, the Joslin facility is state-of-the-art. I'm led past an eye institute, a pediatrics unit, laboratories for basic and clinical research, a library, and a gym—which reminds me of the empty one I saw at the Mallory clinic in Mississippi. Only this one is bustling, with patients putting the treadmills and other apparatus through their paces. I peer through the window, and a petite gray-haired woman hoisting up tiny dumbbells grins at me. This is now their social context; weights and cardio are their new canasta.

Joslin trumpets diabetes-patient education, but so does everyone. The difference here is that the trumpet's blare is the opening rather than the closing note. Education means more than handing patients a brochure, a video, and a drug prescription. New Joslin patients spend an hour with an endocrinologist. Then they spend an hour with another specialist, such as a dietitian, a diabetes educator, an exercise physiologist, or a nurse practitioner. This concerted effort usually results in improved blood sugar control.

Alas, the Joslin Diabetes Center is an exception. Most doctors don't *want* to shuffle needy patients out the door, but one way to offset reduced fees is to see more patients. The best way to see more patients is to fit examination rooms with revolving doors, figuratively speaking. Yet studies have found that the bigger drawback is the reduced feeling of autonomy among doctors. "Our results suggest that when managed care (or other influences) erode professional autonomy, the result is a highly negative impact on physician career satisfaction," wrote the authors of one study. This is particularly worrisome regarding diabetes. Detailed explanations of diets and physical fitness regimens might be perceived by some doctors as going the extra mile, and thus not worth the trouble. Especially if they don't think the patient will follow the advice.

That mind-set doesn't materialize from thin air. "Part of that reflects the way services are reimbursed in our health care system," says Dr. Stafford. "Doing a procedure or prescribing a medication is much more efficient at bringing in dollars than sitting down and talking to a patient. The reluctance to educate the patient may exist on its own, but it's reinforced by how our health care is structured."

THEN AGAIN, MORE face time with a doctor won't help anyway if the person wearing the white coat doesn't recommend the proper course of treatment.

Dr. Berkowitz recalls an episode that illustrates the degree of institutional confusion reigning where diet meets diabetes. "I was asked to give a lecture on diabetes at a hospital trying to raise money for care, and for lunch they served salmon glazed with sugar," he says. "Can you imagine? I'm giving a lecture on diabetes prevention, and that's what they served."

Unglazed salmon ranks among the healthiest foods a diabetic can eat, packed with protein and healthy omega-3 fatty acids, with nary a carb in sight. I eat it all the time. Even coated with sugar, salmon still amounts to a better choice than serving, say, baked rigatoni with low-fat mozzarella. But it makes no sense for those charged with leading the fight against diabetes to sweeten up a healthy food, one that's tasty without it.

The institutional ignorance about diabetes isn't limited to U.S. shores. Ron Raab, past vice president of the International Diabetes Foundation (IDF), recalls attending a breakfast hosted by Diabetes Australia, their version of the ADA, as part of World Diabetes Day. Along with presenting various diabetes talks, the organization had the chance to offer industry experts and politicians a glimpse of what diabetics should be eating for breakfast. "The first course was freshly squeezed orange juice," Raab recalls. "So that's about 22 grams of sugar per eight ounces. The next course included a variety of cereals, such as Kellogg's Corn Flakes. The third course was from the bakery—various breads, such as fruit loaf toast and baguettes."

The common denominator: all major sources of carbs, whose overconsumption can lead to diabetes. Such meal planning is insane, but it was just a warm-up. Says Raab: "They called the next course a 'hot plate.' They threw in a few eggs and some grilled tomatoes, but there were also pine nut pancakes with wild honey. I guess the thinking was, Hey, if it's 'wild,' then it's healthy for diabetics, right?"

By the time Raab tallied all the carbs being served by Diabetes Australia, it came to 200 to 250 grams per person—for one meal! For comparison, a stress test administered by doctors to unmask impaired glucose tolerance, prediabetes, and diabetes contains 75 carb grams. I asked Diabetes Australia what their recommended daily carb intake is for someone with diabetes, and they said they don't have one, that it's specific to every diabetic. That's both true and a cop-out. Of course no one number applies to every diabetic, but the messaging should use percentages and ranges to steer all diabetics in the right direction: fewer carbs and less sugar than nondiabetics.

"Bacon and eggs would have been a much healthier breakfast for diabetics," Raab says. Yet this classic American fare has been witch-hunted by health care professionals because of its fat content, which is mistaken for the real enemy of the overweight and diabetic: sugar. The problem isn't the bacon and eggs; it's the hash browns, toast, and orange juice accompanying them, not to mention the table sugar sprinkled into the coffee used to wash it all down.

I had my own brush with this Orwellian approach to diabetes nutrition during an overnight stay at Lehigh Valley Hospital—Cedar Crest, near where I used to live. Admitted for something unrelated to my prediabetes, I picked up the bedside menu and then placed an order with the hospital cafeteria: marinated seared chicken with a side of broccoli and a diet lemonade. That's a healthy dinner for a prediabetic or anyone, for that matter.

The next morning, I placed a breakfast order of sliced peaches, scrambled eggs and sausage—another solid meal for a diabetic, even if it did contain fruit.

"I'm sorry, but that item's not recommended for your diet," said the pleasant woman on the other end of the line. I had told the doctors that I was prediabetic. I was impressed that this information had been conveyed to the cafeteria.

But I was also confused. "What, the peaches?" I asked.

"No, the sausage."

Diabetes is a disease of carbohydrate metabolism. Sausage contains no carbs. Zero. The peaches, in contrast, had 15 such grams.

For lunch, I decided to conduct an impromptu experiment. I scanned the menu with an eye toward cobbling together the worst possible meal I could think of for someone with prediabetes. Surely this unhealthy order would be struck down as it parted my lips. I asked for a side of potato salad (15 carb grams), followed by rice and beans (45 grams) and angel food cake (15 grams) for dessert. I also asked for a regular Coke (45 grams).

The woman told me the Coke was off-limits. She asked if Diet Coke was okay. But everything else, all 75 grams of it, passed muster.

Isn't it risky to take a different approach than what experts, doctors, and even hospital cafeterias might be recommending? Not necessarily, once you realize that for many doctors, interacting with diabetic patients is a charade. They start with the assumption that preventing the transition from prediabetes or early-stage diabetes to a more advanced version is a losing proposition. The expectation is failure. They think the question is when, not if, that will happen. When I interviewed Dr. Deeb in his capacity as an ADA spokesman, he told me that he sees too many doctors and patients conspiring *not* to take care of their diabetes.

Conspire struck me as an odd word choice in that context. I asked him to elaborate.

He explained, "Let's say you come to see me and I say, 'Your blood sugar is up, and you need to do this, that, and the other thing. In response you say, 'No no no, doc—let's not do that. I'll become more active, I'll lose weight, I'll eat healthier.' And I say, 'Okay, fine, I'll see you in three months.' Well, the time passes, here you are again, and nothing's better. I say, 'No, this isn't working. I need to start you on medicine.' You're like, 'No no no, doc, give me three more months.'

"See how I've conspired with you to *not* take care of you? My take is, Let me take care of you, and if things improve, nothing says I can't take away your medicine."

That seldom happens.

The problem is the carb load overwhelming the metabolic system. Why not suggest a reduction in the harmful influence in the first place? The current approach is akin to offering sleeping pills to an insomniac with a ten-cups-a-day coffee habit. After taking these drugs, the coffee-drinking insomniac wakes up feeling sluggish and needs more coffee to kick-start his or her day. Two balancing "medications" are being used to establish a falsely normal equilibrium. The solution is to drink less coffee, thereby removing both influences.

I'm not saying that this lifestyle message is an easy sell to diabetics. After all, cigarettes contain as many as eight different carcinogens and up to six thousand chemicals, and yet many Americans continue lighting up, knowing that smoking may kill them one day. It says so right on the label, a warning not found on a twelve-ounce can of soda, whose thirteen teaspoons of sugar may also be deadly when habitually consumed.

Even if the message is delivered that eating two Double Quarter Pounders with cheese, fries, and a sugar-laden soda every day lays a fast track to type 2 diabetes, many people will continue dining drive-through style and slugging down sugary sodas. Our society has many bad habits, some harder to break than others. But the message needs to be conveyed more effectively, rather than just telling people that eating *the way they should be eating anyway* is too difficult, and exercising every day *like they should be doing anyway* is too difficult. Of course they give up quickly! Failure is the expectation.

Instead of adequately promoting the simple solution, too many diabetes experts and doctors look for ever more complicated fixes to a problem that will never be solved with a pill or a scalpel.

DOCTORS DON'T MAKE a habit of deliberately withholding the correct dietary information. The problem is that doctors, by and large, aren't well versed in nutrition themselves. For many diseases, that wouldn't be a calamity. True, an unhealthy diet can weaken the immune system, raising the risk of various ills. But many ailments, from staph infections and HIV to Parkinson's and Huntington's diseases aren't actually caused by what a person orders for dinner over long periods of time.

In contrast, type 2 diabetes, which is caused by diet, inactivity, and genetics—as well as the weight gain that often results—is another story. How can doctors address a sloth-and-carbohydrate-created disease, given that so many of them know so little about nutrition and the most beneficial forms of exercise? "Our medical establishment is set up to treat disease, not prevent it," explained Susan M. Kleiner, Ph.D., R.D., a sports nutritionist based in Mercer Island, Washington, in a *Men's Health* article I wrote. "First-year med students rank nutrition among their top priorities. Yet by graduation, it doesn't even make the list. That's because it's not emphasized."

This lack of nutritional knowledge isn't a new problem in the medical community. In 1902, a year before the Wright Brothers powered the first flight, a professor named W. Gilman Thompson was imploring medical schools to make teaching the nutritional sciences a priority. Born in 1856, Thompson received his medical degree from Columbia and studied in London and Berlin before joining a group of New York University rebel-physicians who left to start Cornell University's medical college. Thompson served on the faculty for eighteen years, authoring a book on diet and disease along the way. His critique is as relevant today as it was more than a hundred years ago:

> The subject of the dietetic treatment of disease has not received the attention in medical literature which it deserves, and it is to be regretted that in the curriculum of medical colleges it is usually either omitted or is disposed of in one or two brief lectures at the end of a course in therapeutics. One cannot fail to be impressed with the meager notice given to the necessity of feeding patients properly, and the subject is usually dismissed with brief and indefinite phrases such as: "the value of nutritious diet requires more mention," "a proper but restricted diet is recommended," or "the patient should be carefully fed."

After Thompson's diatribe, nutrition did gain traction in medical schools for a while. This was in part because many diseases of the day resulted from dietary deficiencies and could be cured by rectifying them. Rickets, caused by vitamin D deficiency, was no match for infant foods fortified with that vitamin. Scurvy, caused by severe and chronic vitamin C deficiency, suffered a similar fate. So did pellagra, through the use of supplemental niacin; goiter, once iodine deficiency became easily remedied; and xerophthalmia, which had been caused by deficiency in vitamin A.

The discovery of these deficiency-defeating vitamins and trace minerals gave birth to an entirely new field: clinical nutrition, the science of how nutrients interact with our bodies and their role in keeping us healthy. Medical students began receiving more-vigorous training in the nutritional sciences. Textbooks were rife with information on carbohydrate chemistry, metabolism, and related topics.

The Golden Age of Nutrition, as it came to be known, would lose its luster in the 1950s. After all, dietary deficiencies were mostly solved; thanks to improvements in technology, foods could now be fortified with whatever nutrients they lacked. To the victor went the spoils, as these products could be transported to where people could consume them. Satisfied that it knew what it needed to know about the intersection of food and the human body, the U.S. medical establishment turned its attention elsewhere. Medical curricula followed suit.

At the same time, large-scale farming created cheaper food. Cheaper food meant larger meals. A disease of dietary excess, not deficiency, began creeping across America's medical landscape. As the population grew, both in census figures and waist size, doctors were in no position to counsel diabetic patients on the need to manage their diet because they themselves lacked nutritional expertise. A survey found that by the late 1950s, only 20 percent of U.S. medical schools were devoting as much as a single course to nutrition. The subject was usually shoehorned ad hoc into other classes, no doubt diminishing its importance in students' eyes. *Hey, this is an afterthought* was the message.

In 1985 the Food and Nutrition Board of the National Research Project, part of the National Academy of Sciences, surveyed one-third of all medical schools in the United States. The goal was to gauge how effectively they were teaching the science of nutrition. The survey asked if students were being told of the latest breakthroughs, and if those students were learning how to convey this information to their future patients. The expert panel found a continuation of the decades-long tendency for nutrition to receive short shrift relative to other subjects in medical schools. The final book-thick report was blunt: "The committee concluded that nutrition education programs in U.S. medical schools are largely inadequate to meet the present and future demands of the medical profession."

The panel also recommended that specific dietary topics be included in medical school curricula. These included "energy balance, role of specific nutrients and dietary components, nutrition in the life cycle, nutritional assessment, protein-energy malnutrition, the role of nutrition in disease prevention and treatment, and risks from poor dietary practices stemming from individual, social, and cultural diversity."

Every one of those topics bears directly on type 2 diabetes.

DESPITE THE FOOD and Nutrition Board's entreaties, little progress has been made educating apprentice doctors about nutrition from 1985 until today, even as type 2 diabetes has galloped past all efforts at corralling it. In 2006 University of North Carolina researchers published a study in the *American Journal of Clinical Nutrition* based on surveys of all 126 accredited U.S. medical schools. A mere 30 percent of them were requiring students to take a dedicated nutrition course. Fewer than a third of the schools were requiring the twenty-five-hour minimum of nutritional instruction recommended by the National Academy of Sciences. Eighty-eight percent of the instructors surveyed said students were being underserved with nutritional science. "The amount of nutrition education in medical schools remains inadequate," concluded the authors. I can't think of any major disease benefiting more from this oversight than type 2 diabetes.

The net result is a surprising lack of awareness about the interplay between nutrition and diabetes found in even those at the highest levels of the medical establishment—like the presidency of the American Academy of Family Physicians (AAFP). Founded in 1947, the AAFP is among the largest medical organizations in the country, boasting a membership of some 94,000 names, roughly 11 percent of the physicians and medical students in the United States.

During a 2007 interview with the AAFP's then-president James King, M.D., a family physician in Selmer, Tennessee, I asked him how to eat properly as a prediabetic so that I could inform others in the pages of *Men's Health*. "I tell diabetic patients to consume more carbohydrates—mainly from fruits and vegetables, not from simple sugars and starches—while decreasing the amount of meat and fat in their diet," he said.

The average American takes in 2,157 calories a day, according to recent U.S. government survey data. Fifty percent of those calories come from carbs, 33 percent from fat, 15 percent from protein, and 2 percent from alcohol. That works out to about 262 grams of carbohydrates a day. Divided among three meals a day, as Dr. King suggests eating, leaves 87 carb grams per meal. Each of these meals contains 12 grams *more* than the amount of carbs administered for a metabolic stress test. Mind you, any such test is designed to be an exceptional scenario, not an everyday occurrence. To test the wings of an airplane, engineers flex them to 150 percent of the worst imaginable scenario ever to be duplicated in the skies, to see if their structural integrity will hold. The test lasts three seconds. They don't run it over and over for years and then load the plane with passengers once the wings are so fatigued that they'll snap off at the first bump of turbulence.

The irony is that Dr. King and the AAFP are suggesting that meat (i.e., protein) and fat be reduced from the average amounts now consumed. To keep calories adequate, that requires even more carbs; no getting around it. So the diabetic patient, whose carb intake is already higher than levels used to run a stress test, is being told to consume . . . more carbs!

Later in the same conversation, I asked Dr. King if spacing out meals should be a consideration for diabetics and prediabetics. Not really, he said, adding: "What we recommend when we start treating diabetes is that patients eat two meals a day, along with one smaller meal. Eat when you're hungry, and eat the right foods when you do."

In prediabetes and early-stage diabetes, when insulin levels are high, your blood sugar drops, making you hungry. So the recommendation from Dr. King and the AAFP is to reach for exactly the sort of foods that will trigger yet another insulin spike and blood sugar crash. Diabetics need to be eating before they become hungry, not after, at which point it's too late.

Apart from the mental impairment and health risks posed by chronically low blood sugar, the hypoglycemic state—usually defined as blood glucose below 70 mg/dL—is when you're most prone to blow your diet. You feel half-awake, a bad time for self-discipline. When researchers at

Florida State University performed tests of self-control on men, the lowest blood sugar readings corresponded with the moments of weakest willpower. However, that willpower doubled after a glass of lemonade, which gave the brain a quick fuel burst. Unfortunately, lemonade—exactly the kind of sugary antidote that experience tells someone they should reach for in that situation—will trigger another blood sugar spike and then crash.

THE U.S. HEALTH care system is structured so that once a patient makes the transition from prediabetes to type 2 diabetes, a dietitian can enter the picture. But only if invited. "Unfortunately, when the dietitian is interjected often depends on the doctor," says Angela Ginn-Meadow, R.D., L.D.N., C.D.E., an American Dietetic Association spokeswoman I interviewed. "I've seen patients who have never seen a dietitian or a diabetes educator despite having been diagnosed with diabetes for ten or twenty years. It depends. Some physicians refer the patient to nutritional counseling; others say, 'Well, just cut out the sweets or watch what you eat or lose the weight.' It takes the patient being the champion and saying, 'I think I need more help.'" Typically it doesn't occur to a patient under the care of a trusted medical doctor to seek out a qualified dietitian on his or her own. Why would they?

As a result, a person's first encounter with a dietitian often coincides with a hospitalization because of hyperglycemia. By then a crisis has developed, whereas diet changes are most effective as an ounce of prevention. What's worse, this might be the only meeting the patient will ever have with a dietitian. It doesn't help that most insurance companies don't cover nutritional counseling for prediabetics, despite prediabetes being the last chance to forestall the onset of what is a dietary disease. This system seems more than a little backward, like fastening your seat belt after a crash.

The actual advice being given to diabetics by mainstream dietitians is as perplexing as its timing. The American Dietetic Association, as much as anyone, determines what Americans eat and drink. Operating since 1917, with more than seventy thousand members, this *other* ADA dwarfs the other U.S. professional nutrition societies. It also boasts a long list of corporate sponsors, including Coca-Cola, Pepsico, Kellogg's, General Mills, and Mars. Many of the best-selling products of these companies are loaded with carbohydrates, which makes you wonder: What is the ADA's perspective on the relationship between carbs and diabetes?

The association includes the Diabetes Care and Education Dietetic Practice Group (DCE), a panel of professionals seeking to promote quality diabetes care and education. According to the executive summary of the ADA's nutrition practice guidelines for adults with type 1 or type 2 diabetes, dietitians who work with diabetics should follow macronutrient guidelines outlined for healthy adults in the Dietary Reference Intakes. Think of these as the commandments of the government's nutrition bible. In a broad recommendation for average Americans, the U.S. government calls for carbs to represent 45 to 65 percent of total energy intake. The top of that range is outrageously overboard for a diabetic—you might as well be receiving dietary recommendations from Betty Crocker.

The implication is that whatever carb load works for someone with normal glucose metabolism should work equally well for someone whose body can't handle the sugar that most carbs become after digestion. This is the nonsensical message drummed into the heads of dietitians over their four years of training. Never mind that a huge swath of the population can't handle that many carbs.

Doctors convey this same dietary advice to their patients and then blame them when the treatment fails to manage or reverse diabetes. "I was one of those jaded doctors in a busy clinic who would say 'Go do this' and feel like my patients would never do it," says Eric C. Westman, M.D., director of the Duke Lifestyle Medicine Clinic. "My initial judgment—probably a lot of doctors' judgment—was, 'They're not doing what I say,' rather than, 'Maybe what we're telling them is wrong.'"

4

METABOLIC MYSTERIES

There are probably more than half a million diabetics in the United States. Therefore, it is proper at the present time to devote attention not alone to treatment, but still more, as in the campaign against typhoid fever, to prevention. The results may not be quite so striking or as immediate, but they are sure to come and to be important.

—*Elliott P. Joslin, M.D.,* Journal of the American Medical Association, *January 8, 1921*

The decades of decay and slow-motion death that I witnessed at my father's bedside came from high blood glucose and the resulting blood vessel damage. Sadly, it was preventable. Yet diabetes was once a short-and-sweet death sentence with no reprieve. The disease was so unusual, so hard to explain, so impossible to treat, and so horrific in its consequences that it might have seemed like the devil's work. One report, written in 1893 by a third-year Harvard Medical School student assigned to a twenty-six-year-old patient named Mary Higgins, made it sound like an exorcism might be the only Rx. "Her hair [had] dropped out," he wrote. "Her strength and flesh melted away from her body . . . [she had an] odour of acetone to her breath and with the professor of chemistry I demonstrated acetone and diacetic acid."

That student, Elliott Proctor Joslin, was born in Oxford, Massachusetts, in June 1869, a time when the source of diabetes, let alone its cure, was mysterious. For those more inclined to medical rather than supernatural explanations, the liver, not the pancreas, was the prime suspect back then. It wasn't until the late 1880s, when two German scientists noticed that a dog developed diabetes after having its pancreas removed, that the source of the disease was properly attributed for the first time.

Joslin came from a privileged background. His father was heir to a family fortune made from leather tanning, and his mother, Sarah, also came from wealth. Their son's attention was drawn to medicine rather than building a business, and he became obsessed with understanding and treating diabetes. Armed with a Harvard medical degree, he crossed the Atlantic to study with some of Europe's leading blood sugar experts. After returning home, he fashioned America's first diabetes clinic in his parents' Boston town house at 81 Bay State Road.

Patients didn't show up just from the far reaches of the United States and Europe; they were already inside the brownstone. His aunt Helen had already been diagnosed as a diabetic; in 1899, it was his mother's turn. Whether it was Mary Higgins (the first entry), his mother (the eighth), or some other victim he encountered in the examining room, Dr. Joslin would record their plight in a series of large accounting ledgers. At the behest of a mentor, he also pored through diabetes case studies going back seventy-five years at Massachusetts General Hospital. Dr. Joslin came to realize that no progress had been made against the disease in at least three-quarters of a century.

Aside from a few prescient observers, doctors back then had yet to link what we now call type 2 diabetes with obesity. Life insurance companies, who had money at stake, also noted that obese people often became diabetic and died prematurely as a result. Employing rudimentary statistical analysis before it became a science, Dr. Joslin paired actuarial data with his own observations, concluding, "Diabetes . . . is largely a penalty of obesity, and the greater the obesity, the more likely is Nature to enforce it."

Given his family history of diabetes, Dr. Joslin obsessed over his own weight. Dieting and exercising with great discipline kept him under 170 pounds and his BMI at a rail-thin 21. It was an example he expected his diabetic patients to follow, counseling them to remain 10 percent under what would normally be considered their ideal body weight. Nor did he sugarcoat the truth for overweight diabetics, writing, "It is generally prudent and always far more effective to say to the patient: 'You are too fat,' than cautiously to remark: 'You are a trifle obese.'" Even his mother found herself on a diet low in calories and carbohydrates, which produced a diabetic remission, at least for a while.

"Implicit in some of that early work was the notion that you could remit the type 2s," says Dr. Barnett. "That made him optimistic and hopeful, although some people called it whistling in the dark." Alas, Mrs. Joslin's death in 1913 is recorded in the ledgers, too.

The type 1s weren't so lucky. The human immune system is designed to ward off viruses, bacteria, and other invaders, but sometimes it doesn't know when to stop the counterattack. As a result, healthy tissues are destroyed. Sometimes the victims of this friendly fire are the beta cells of the pancreas. They can no longer produce insulin, which is the defining characteristic of type 1 diabetes. This autoimmune response occurs most often during childhood or adolescence, which explains the disease's former name, juvenile diabetes. That nomenclature is obsolete because type 2 now strikes children so often. For the same reason, type 2 is no longer called adult-onset diabetes.

This division of diabetes types was noticed as far back as 500 B.C., according to a group of medical historians writing in a 2008 issue of *Dartmouth Medicine*: "Sushruta . . . an early exponent of Ayurvedic medicine—observed that the urine of . . . patients [who passed too much] tasted like honey, and was sticky to the touch, and attracted ants. He even described two forms of the disease—one occurring in older, obese individuals and the other in young individuals who did not live long after the diagnosis."

Diabetes mellitus, the full name of diabetes, combines the Greek word for "siphon" with the Latin word for "honey." Sweet urine.

Before insulin became widely available in 1923, type 1 children seldom lived for more than a year. Any sugar entering their body was left unregulated, leading to the rapid buildup of acid. The only controls left were the calorie and the carb, and the Joslin method was miserly with each. Patients whose blood was toxic would be limited to drinking liquids such as water, tea, and bouillon for three days. This was a temporary fast, not the "starvation diet" that some claimed. But patients who were already thin from excessive urination grew thinner still. Once the toxic acidosis was brought under control, Dr. Joslin would titrate calories back into the diet.

"Allowing these patients to become even thinner than they already were seemed bizarre to many observers," says Dr. Barnett. "But consider the alternative: Eat up to satisfy your appetite and die in the process."

Preinsulin, the typical Dr. Elliot Joslin Diabetic Diet for noncritical patients was 75 percent fat, consisting mostly of meat, cheese, and cream. The latter in particular helped with satiety. Carbs contributed only about 5 percent of total calories, thanks to Dr. Joslin cutting out bread, fruit, milk, and "white" vegetables such as potatoes, corn, and rice. Red and green vegetables remained, but only in moderation.

His extreme approach prompted a firestorm of criticism, but Dr. Joslin was a contrarian by nature. A great-grandfather seven times removed was John Proctor, immortalized in Arthur Miller's play *The Crucible*. Proctor had spoken out against the Salem witch trials and was in turn then accused of witchcraft. He was convicted and hanged in 1692.

If you think the dietary adjustments required by diabetes amount to a test of will now, imagine what it was like before insulin. An Italian diabetes expert from the late nineteenth century, Catoni, locked away his patients to keep them from cheating. To ensure that his own patients wouldn't be sneaking chocolate cake in violation of his regimen, Dr. Joslin admitted them to a special metabolic ward at New England Deaconess Hospital in Boston, with nurse practitioners working the room like so many Florence Nightingales. "Wandering nurses" they were called, for their penchant not only to tend to the metabolic ward but also to venture outside of it, making private house calls, often lasting for days, to educate diabetics and their families on the vagaries of insulin vis-à-vis diet and exercise, and on how to prevent insulin reactions.

Dr. Joslin's radical Rx worked. Well, sort of. Dietary restrictions so drastic might extend a patient's life an extra year, maybe eighteen months. Critics thought diabetics should enjoy some semblance of normalcy during whatever remained of their lives, rather than try to eke out a few more months through asceticism. The denial-versus-indulgence debate has often had a religious tenor, perhaps because it pits those tendencies in a life-and-death struggle. When I met with him in Boston, Dr. Barnett used the analogy of John Calvin and Pope Paul III, casting Dr. Joslin as Calvin, the reformist French theologian, and the U.S. diabetes establishment of the mid-twentieth century as the Roman Catholic Church. "[Dr. Joslin's] pleading to live an organized life, in the age in which he preached it, did not go over well with the group who was either over-controlled by their puritanical background, or were so poor in the old country that they wanted to eat [heartily]," said Dr. Barnett.

Some diabetic youths would visit a diabetes camp in New York, but one "wag," as Barnett puts it, would refer to it as Camp Forget. "They'd tell you to just put your diabetes in the umbrella rack when you came there, and eat up," said Dr. Barnett. Leave it to magical insulin to clean up the mess. Dr. Joslin, in contrast, ran boot camps for young diabetics, preparing them for a lifelong battle against an enemy that didn't retreat.

Dr. Barnett describes the Joslin Clinic of old as "a cross between a military unit and a religious order in tone and purpose," and its leader embodied both aspects. With his slight build, hairless pate, and round specs, the Dr. Joslin in old photos looks serene and remote. He reminds me of a Yankee version of Gandhi. In reality, he was a field general, cracking the whip on foot soldiers, who revered and feared him in equal measure. "He built a team, and he needed one," says Dr. Barnett. "He had the triangle of hell to deal with: coma, gangrene, and infection. Can you imagine treating diabetics before antibiotics? It was *awful*." With his wild-eyed demeanor and lengthy conversational footnotes, this delightful chronicler of Dr. Joslin looks and sounds like Peter O'Toole channeling David Foster Wallace. He's prone to start scribbling furiously in his notepad as he speaks, presumably making a note to self.

Staff meetings ended every morning at 8:42 A.M., after which Dr. Joslin saw up to fifteen patients a day. He was as kind to them as he was tough on his staffers. Using a thousand of his own cases, he wrote his first diabetes textbook, *The Treatment of Diabetes*, published fourteen editions ago in 1916. (Subsequent editions have been published under the title *Joslin's Diabetes Mellitus*.) But the self-help manifesto, *A Diabetic Manual for the Mutual Use of Doctor and Patient*, came two years later. "Doctor and Patient" is the key phrase here. He realized that daily management of this disease falls on the patient, not the doctor.

Dr. Joslin hailed insulin as a nearly biblical revelation for diabetics and their caregivers. With this new tool in the kit, calorie reductions could go from Draconian to merely prudent and strict. As the preeminent diabetologist of his era, Dr. Joslin helped lead the way in testing the new drug in his patients. His descriptions of their awakenings from diabetic comas read more like visions than case notes. "I had witnessed so many near resurrections that I realized I was seeing enacted before my very eyes Ezekiel's vision of the valley of dry bones," he wrote, invoking the Old Testament.

Dr. Joslin believed that type 1 diabetics should use insulin to achieve rigorous glucose control. He believed this would help delay and lessen diabetic complications. Yet this view was often reviled, and he along with it, even as it became clear to many in the field that he was right, especially concerning those complications affecting the small blood vessels of the eyes and kidneys. (Although diabetes is a huge risk factor for cardiovascular disease, the benefit of tight glucose control on preventing cardiac arrest is still not an open-and-shut case.) This debate ended in 1993, two decades after Dr. Joslin died at age ninety-two, when the *New England Journal of Medicine* published the results of a large study called the Diabetes Control and Complications Trial. Type 1 diabetics who had undergone intensive glucose-control therapy were found to have less vascular damage to the small blood vessels than diabetics receiving conventional treatment.

ALONG WITH POSSESSING an almost magical potency, insulin is ancient; it was found in organisms whose habitat was the cauldron of primitive life-forms known as primordial soup. Insulin allowed our own earliest ancestors to make a huge evolutionary leap. Their bodies could store fuel, which afforded them time for other pursuits. They could erect family structures, tell stories, and build languages now that they didn't have to hunt and scavenge all day for nourishment. Insulin helped make us human.

Insulin helps the body metabolize the sugar in the blood, which is called glucose. This blood sugar can come from diet, but the liver and kidneys can also produce it. What isn't needed for energy can also be stored in muscle tissue and the liver. This stored form is called glycogen. But because storage space is limited, at a certain point, the liver begins turning excess glucose into triglycerides, which often become body fat. The human body has evolved such that it possesses a very low capacity to store carbs but a very high capacity to store fat. This phenomenon is evident in buffet lines across the heartland.

"That's in a relatively healthy person," says Jeff S. Volek, Ph.D., R.D., associate professor of kinesiology at the University of Connecticut. "Even before glycogen levels fill up, people with insulin resistance dispose of carbohydrates by converting the majority of them to fat." That's one reason why the heavy become still heavier, even if they pass on the second helpings.

Nearly every cell in the body can take up and use glucose as fuel, and blood travels everywhere in the body, making it the ideal transporter of glucose to far-flung destinations. But how does the glucose know where to go? A messenger hormone called insulin escorts it. Certain tissues in the body attract insulin; their surface is lined with welcoming receptors. Receptors are proteins, but think of them more as magnets. Most of these insulin receptors are located in muscle tissue, a function of muscle's large size and metabolic activity.

The system is designed to work so that after you eat a meal, the pancreas releases insulin in an amount proportional to whatever the glucose load happens to be. Insulin arrives at receptors and is recognized as such, and cells know what to do in response: absorb glucose from the bloodstream. So your blood glucose never shoots too high. As this process unfolds, a feedback loop signals the pancreas to produce less insulin, to keep the messengers home. So your blood glucose never falls too low, either. The normal blood sugar response to a meal is a slow rise followed by a reasonable drop.

Insulin resistance occurs when insulin tries but fails to bind with receptors, and glucose is left stranded. Instead of taking five units of insulin to produce a certain amount of energy from glucose, it's now taking your body, say, twenty. All the pancreas knows is that insulin isn't doing its job, so it keeps secreting more and more, to little avail.

This creates an energy crisis for each cell, not to mention for your entire body. To use a crude analogy: Imagine oil tankers sailing from port to port loaded with oil (glucose) that needs to be loaded onto smaller boats (insulin) for transport to shore. But once the oil has been loaded onto the smaller vessels, these boats bounce off the docks, unable to land. Thus the raw material never makes it to shore, and the factories in town sit idle. The crude oil can't be delivered. Productivity halts.

Unfortunately the lifestyle choices causing insulin resistance—not exercising, indulging a sweet tooth, and eating too much in general—trigger a feedback loop. Particularly if you don't exercise, those excess carbs will cause blood sugar to spike and then crash, at which point the body bellies up for another round of sugar.

Since your body is dumping glucose into boats that can't land, it must find another fuel source. An alternative is fat, which can be burned for energy as long as oxygen and mitochondria, the parts of the cells that contain fat-burning enzymes, are present. Luckily, only a few places in the entire body lack oxygen, mitochondria, or both. Red blood cells don't possess those tiny power plants, so it may be no coincidence that glucose floats around in blood. The lens of the eye and a remote area of the kidneys also depend solely on glucose. But that's about it.

It should hardly come as a surprise, then, that diabetes consistently attacks these parts of the body. The kidneys are one of only two organs capable of producing glucose from noncarb sources such as protein, the liver being the other.

So glucose is essential for life, and it usually comes from carbs. Wouldn't we cease to function if we didn't consume enough carbs?

Consider: In the early 1900s, a pair of Arctic explorers, Vilhjalmur Stefansson and Rudolph M. Anderson, marveled at not only the carnivorous diets but also the robust health of Eskimos. So upon returning from their expedition, the two men embarked upon a meat-only diet. The resulting macronutrient ratio amounted to 75 to 85 percent fat and 1 to 2 percent carbohydrates. Protein made up the balance. At the end of what was a yearlong experiment, they were alive and well, although perhaps a bit grumpy.

To find out how they survived, I spent a day at Dr. Westman's Duke clinic on my way back from the ADA conference in New Orleans. As befits someone who grew up in the cheese state of Wisconsin, the good doctor puts patients needing to shed extra pounds, manage diabetes, or both on a low-carb diet. To great effect, I might add. He's fascinated by which organs actually need glucose—not which ones use it when it's available. As I trail him into his office, my gaze is drawn to a homemade anatomy-chart-turned-schematic on one wall. The names of bodily organs are computer-printed on pieces of paper. This anatomy chart is proportional rather than representational; each cutout reflects the energy requirement of that organ, rather than its shape or size. I see that the liver sucks up as much glucose as the brain. "Pretty much everything can run on fat," says the Stanford grad, noting the exceptions mentioned before—red blood cells, retina, and a remote region of the kidneys.

The assumption has been that dietary carbohydrates must provide 130 grams of glucose per day for the brain and central nervous system to function fully. But Dr. Westman insists that the liver and kidneys could produce more than enough glucose from protein to supply that amount, which explains why those Eskimos, and the explorers who found them, could live on only meat. No, I can't imagine any sane non-Eskimo wanting to follow the Eskimo Diet, which is a product of their unique habitat. But the wall schematic is illuminating nonetheless. Everyone, from Gatorade and General Mills, to the corn lobby and dietetic organizations, keeps telling us that we need *all* these carbs, and that eating them gives us *all* this energy.

We're being implored to eat them for reasons that have little to do with any sort of internal need. I bought into their sales pitch, and I write about this stuff for a living. The truth is, we don't need all those carbs, and they don't give us all that energy. In fact we don't need nearly as many carbs as we are implored to consume by everything from government guidelines to television commercials. "The Western diet is far too high in carbohydrates," says the IDF's Raab. The metabolic system of the average human being was designed to run on some debatable fraction of that amount.

The solution to the type 2 diabetes epidemic isn't force-feeding the hard-core Atkins approach to everyone who's either a diabetic or at risk of becoming one—although that approach, if followed, would produce better results than the approach we take now. But the solution isn't the status quo approach of the diabetes industry, either. The evidence against that is prima facie. Just look at what amounts to an epidemiological study including the entire U.S. population, which makes the conventional wisdom look increasingly unwise.

Part of the solution for America's obesity and diabetes epidemics is a diet lower in carbs—and less internal insulin production as a result—and a higher intake of protein and healthy fats. This will result in much better glucose control. But you won't hear that recommendation from most diabetes organizations and experts.

THE ELEPHANT IN the room when it comes to type 2 diabetes is the beer-belly/love-handles factor. Yes, obesity is a driving force behind the diabetes epidemic, and the most conspicuous factor. A strong association exists: Many type 2 diabetics weigh too much, and many heavyset individuals will become type 2 diabetics, if they haven't already. But which factor is the chicken and which is the egg prompts a lot of back-and-forth among diabetes and obesity experts.

Perhaps the question should be framed this way: Does something else cause both obesity *and* type 2 diabetes? Think of diabetes and weight gain as separate manifestations of insulin resistance. Being overweight skyrockets the odds of also having high blood sugar, but it's more an association than a cause and an effect. Weight loss provides one of the best antidotes to type 2 diabetes and prediabetes, not necessarily because the weight gain caused blood sugar to rise. More likely, exercise, calorie reduction, carb cutting, and other strategies that lead to sustainable weight loss also heighten insulin sensitivity. The distinction is partly semantic, but it makes you think about what's causing your body to spin out of control in the first place. Improvement matters here, not swimsuit-model perfection.

"Researchers find that even a relatively small loss of weight can have a significant benefit in blood sugar control, regardless of how you lose the weight," says Andrew J. Ahmann, M.D., medical director of the Oregon Health and Science University Diabetes Center. In fact, the Diabetes Prevention Program found that for each kilogram of body weight lost, a person's risk of developing type 2 diabetes dropped by 16 percent!

How does insulin resistance make so many people obese? As I mentioned, when the condition begins taking hold, the body responds by pumping out even more insulin. Calories become trapped in fat cells instead of stored in muscle, and the metabolic system finds itself in a quandary. With so much insulin present, fat can't be broken down for energy. Cells can't absorb much glucose, either, with insulin being ineffectual.

Insulin-resistant cells can no longer gain access to the energy they need, so they conserve what remains. The body begins telling the brain: *Don't do any exercise, and, please, would you eat more?* As these people gain weight, the standard approach is to tell them: *Get your tail off of the sofa and go for a jog! And whatever you do, stop eating!* "This usually fails because their internal signaling is telling them to do the opposite," says Jay Wortman, M.D., senior medical advisor for the First Nations and Inuit Health Branch of Health Canada. "It takes a lot of willpower to overcome those signals."

Type 2 diabetes and obesity aren't interchangeable. Nor does one necessarily cause the other. The overlay of type 2 diabetes and obesity is a Venn diagram. Based on his experiments, Gerald M. Reaven, M.D., endocrinologist and professor (active) emeritus in medicine at the Stanford University School of Medicine, has discovered that one-third of all obese people are *not* insulin resistant. At the same time, 10 to 15 percent of the insulin resistant are not overweight, according to Donald W.

Bowden, Ph.D., director of the Center for Diabetes Research at Wake Forest University School of Medicine. However, that percentage soars for certain groups. An African American woman who's not overweight, for example, still has a 50 percent chance of showing insulin resistance.

Unfortunately, being of normal weight or even skinny and insulin resistant is accompanied by the same metabolic cluster bomb—hyperglycemia, low HDL, hypertension, etc.—ticking inside the heavy and insulin resistant. No wonder being thin offers no immunity from diabetes or heart disease. "People are eating a diet that predisposes them to diabetes, and that diet also causes a lot of people to gain weight," says Dr. Wortman. "There are overweight people who don't have metabolic problems, and normal-weight people who do have these problems. That's telling us that weight gain isn't the underlying cause of diabetes. Something else causes both, and it's our diet."

"There's no textbook body type for diabetics anymore," says Dr. Berkowitz. "It's become harder to diagnose as a result." Look overseas, where diabetes is rampant. In Asia, diabetics tend not to be as heavy as they are in the United States. According to a 2006 article in the *New York Times*, "a 5-foot-9 Japanese man who weighs 156 pounds—and who may never develop the sort of belly that is a warning sign for the disease—is twice as likely as a white man that size to become diabetic."

Of the 224 million adults living in the United States, more than 80 million have insulin resistance severe enough to make them at least prediabetic. The 8 to 12 million of them who aren't overweight are a metabolic mystery with a counterintuitive condition. As such, their ranks may well exceed what these calculations suggest. One limiting factor is that people in this group tend to die prematurely, despite their healthy appearance. When a heart attack or some other diabetic-type complication kills them prematurely, survivors often ask: "Why him or her? That doesn't make sense."

"Insulin resistance alone is a factor for heart disease," says Wake Forest University's Bowden. "If you don't have diabetes but are insulin resistant—and much of the U.S. population is—you're at increased risk for heart disease. You may also get diabetes, but your heart disease likely will have gotten worse long before that happens."

Says Dr. Wortman: "At first glance, the constellation of metabolic syndrome, type 2 diabetes, and cardiovascular disease don't seem to be obviously connected. Only now we understand that they are. I've come to view type 2 diabetes, metabolic syndrome, and obesity as part of a continuum linked by a common factor, which is insulin resistance."

Insulin sensitivity can vary eightfold between any two individuals, even healthy ones. Biology seldom accommodates a spread so wide. "As it turns out, only 25 percent of the variability can be attributed to differences in body fat," Dr. Reaven told me. "Another 25 percent comes from differences in fitness level. The rest is likely genetic." So the individual who becomes obese through inactivity *and* has a genetic predisposition is likelier than most to become insulin resistant en route to type 2 diabetes.

Many doctors may be botching the treatment of overweight diabetics, but they aren't even looking for insulin resistance in normal-weight individuals like my father and me. And even if they did identify these mystery men and women, many doctors wouldn't know what to do next. After all, the standard advice for diabetics—"You need to lose some weight"—isn't the relevant prescription. That's like telling an infertile couple wanting to conceive that all they need is more Viagra.

THE CORRECT LIFESTYLE changes for addressing diabetes work wonders without pharmaceutical assistance, assuming the disease hasn't taken full control. Specifically, people need to exercise more and consume fewer carbs. "The human body is designed to handle certain forms and amounts of carbohydrate, but not what we're giving it," says Ron Raab, who is president of Insulin for Life, which takes insulin that would otherwise be discarded and redirects it to type 1 diabetics in the less-developed world. "The high-carb advice from the profession itself has created the circumstances for otherwise healthy bodies to break down in response to a diet it was never designed to handle. We're manufacturing type 2 diabetes in the same way we would skin cancer if the guidance was for people to sit on the beach all day, every day."

Diabetes care has become a major profit driver, and business is booming. According to a paper by a researcher at the Stanford University School of Medicine and others, the U.S. spent $12.5 billion on diabetes prescriptions in 2007, surpassed only by sales of cholesterol drugs. That's nearly twice the amount spent in 2001. An August 2010 report issued by industry analysts at Morningstar forecast the global market for diabetes drugs, excluding insulin, to exceed $55 billion by 2019. Yet the pace of this rapidly growing disease will only have accelerated.

Diabetics should be able to enjoy carb foods like nondiabetics do, the official line goes, but they need to make sure to take whatever action is necessary, drugs included, to cause rising blood sugar to ebb. On its Web site, the ADA recommends that diabetics divide their breakfast plate in half and fill one side with starchy foods such as breads, cereals, or potatoes, all of which will be readily converted to sugar in the body. The next step is to halve the empty space and fill one part with fruit, more fast-acting carbs. The remaining (optional) quarter is reserved for a breakfast meat. An egg, arguably the single healthiest food on the planet for diabetics, has no place on this table.

The ADA isn't done carb loading a nation of diabetics, however. They recommend washing it all down with an eight-ounce glass of non-fat or low-fat milk. All told, that's equivalent to eating several candy bars' worth of carbs, providing a feeding frenzy for the disease that the ADA seeks to prevent with its recommendations.

Click on their "Breakfast on the Go" link, and the advice becomes even wackier. Their five suggestions all contain enough fast-acting carbs to start your day off with a blood sugar crash. They actually recommend microwaving half a baked potato and topping it with low-fat cheddar cheese and salsa.

The dietary advice for diabetics is equally misguided on the Web site of the National Institutes of Health (NIH) National Diabetes Information Clearinghouse. They show what they call the Diabetes Food Pyramid, with starches along the bottom, fruits and vegetables on the second floor, and milk and meat on the third floor. Fats and sweets reside at the pinnacle.

"Eat more from the groups at the bottom of the pyramid, and less from the groups at the top," it reads below the pyramid. "Foods from the starches, fruits, vegetables, and milk groups are highest in carbohydrate. They affect your blood glucose levels the most."

"Affect" as in cause to rise, which is what diabetics try to avoid: high blood sugar. The dietary advice for diabetics being dispensed by the highest U.S. medical authorities isn't just contradictory; it's also nonsensical.

Little wonder we're losing this war. "The majority of Americans still think the ideal diet for their health is high in carbohydrate and low in fat," says Raab. "To make a major difference in this diabetes epidemic, switching to a significantly lower-carbohydrate diet [should serve] as the mainstream advice."

When it comes to recommending an effective antidiabetes nutritional strategy, the diabetes establishment may have been closer to the mark in 1921 than it is in 2011. Over the near century during which type 2 diabetes has gone from being a medical oddity to a household name, the ADA has nearly tripled the number of carbs recommended in the average diabetic's diet. To them, sugar isn't the problem. In its most current position statement devoted expressly to carbs and diabetes, the ADA wrote, "[T]here is little evidence that total carbohydrate intake is associated with the development of type 2 diabetes. Rather, a stronger association has been observed between total fat and saturated fat intake and type 2 diabetes."

"The ADA has long recommended this low-fat, high-carbohydrate diet, but that's just about the worst thing you can do if you're insulin resistant," says Dr. Reaven, who is no lightweight, having defined the concept of metabolic syndrome that's now acknowledged worldwide. "It's a horrible idea. The response to more carbohydrate from someone who's insulin resistant is to make more insulin. If you're diabetic, you'll become more hyperglycemic and your triglycerides will go up in response." As a result, the officially sanctioned dietary doctrine will require diabetics to take more drugs to manage their disease.

Spoon-feeding more sugar to a disease whose main symptom is high blood sugar doesn't make a lick of sense. "Would you feed someone who is lactose intolerant . . . lactose?" asks Volek of the University of Connecticut. "Yet we encourage people who are already intolerant of carbs to keep on eating them. It's making them sick and forcing them to use drugs. Only even with aggressive drug therapy, their condition will deteriorate."

If it makes no sense, why are we doing it?

"We tend to be a culture of quick fix-ism when it comes to what people hope for in facing an illness, even a chronic one like type 2 diabetes," says Arthur Caplan, Ph.D., chair of the department of medical ethics at the University of Pennsylvania. "We want to take something for it, and doctors want to supply it. The message is often, 'We've got a pill, I heard it's effective, and, um, sure, you can exercise, but let's move on that pill because there's evidence that it works.'"

When it comes to type 2 diabetes, that mind-set has been a windfall for the pharmaceutical industry, prosthetic-limb makers, and, perhaps, those who breed Seeing Eye dogs. For the rest of us, it's been a disaster.

DOCTORS AND RESEARCHERS have suspected for nearly half a century that hypertension, elevated blood glucose, high triglycerides, low HDL, and belly fat share more in common than being stand-alone risk factors for heart disease and type 2 diabetes. Not coincidentally, where one appears, the others likely lurk. Cops would call them known associates. However, the nature of their relationship has been another long-standing medical mystery. Why do these same problems always seem to crop up together?

Researchers and clinicians alike have sought a conceptual framework that would bring these symptoms under an umbrella. In 1988, Stanford's Gerald Reaven gave a lecture explaining how glucose intolerance, lipid problems, hypertension, and diabetes were part of a single phenomenon. He called it Syndrome X. But Reaven's catchphrase wasn't what shook up the crowd. It was his theory of the underlying cause for all these symptoms—insulin resistance, a concept that had been dismissed as quackery by the medical establishment. This is a recurring theme in the history of U.S. diabetes care: Those who end up being right are usually vilified, ridiculed, or both, often for decades.

Reaven revealed that a person didn't even have to become diabetic for insulin resistance to be harmful. High levels of circulating insulin raise blood pressure and triglycerides while lowering good cholesterol. Heart disease could kill a person before diabetes did. This holistic view had been lacking up to that point; unfortunately, many doctors still haven't taken it to heart. They view diabetes and heart disease as distinct medical problems that pop up together at random. In reality, their kinship is much closer than most people realize.

Not until 1998 did the World Health Organization embrace Reaven's concept, slapping on a fresh coat of paint and labeling virtually the same array of symptoms as metabolic syndrome. Since then other health organizations have accepted the concept as being valid while endeavoring to mark that territory as their own. In 1999, the European Group for the Study of Insulin Resistance made a few minor adjustments to the condition and renamed it insulin resistance syndrome. In 2001, the National Cholesterol Educational Program Adult Treatment Panel III offered a new version that wasn't very different from the old versions, later bringing it into accordance with ADA guidelines. Not to be outdone, the IDF offered its own hair-splitting description of metabolic syndrome in 2005.

The syndrome's name and components can be tweaked endlessly, but it all boils down to the same menace: insulin resistance.

5

COME, SWEET DEATH

f you've ever seen a pancreas up close, you probably weren't impressed. It lacks the dark mystery of the brain, holds none of the allure of the heart. Still, for a squishy-looking glob, the pancreas sure can kill you in a lot of creative ways.

Government statistics will tell you that diabetes is the seventh leading cause of death in the United States. But that ranking is in many ways an illusion. Type 2 diabetes usually covers its tracks by ending a life some other way—a stroke, a heart attack, toxic shock from a gangrenous limb—first. "Diabetes-related complications" they're euphemistically called. A report issued by the American Association of Clinical Endocrinologists found that 60 percent of type 2 diabetics are already saddled with another serious health problem associated with the disease.

"I think everyone in the field would agree that the mortality rate of diabetes drastically underestimates the scope of the problem," says Barry Braun, Ph.D., associate professor at the University of Massachusetts in Amherst, and an expert in the relationship between exercise and insulin resistance.

Diabetes's versatility as a killer came to life for me one day in August when I cracked open Dr. Joslin's old diabetes ledgers in Boston. The handwriting was elegant and exacting; this man was never careless, I suspect. Feeling the worn leather, seeing the faded ink and fingerprints, I could picture the doctor and his patients. At far left were the names. Across each row was medical data such as the patient's age, weight, blood pressure, and date of diagnosis. At the far right was a column listing cause of death. Even though these were all diabetics, the term diabetes mellitus appeared only here and there. Instead, that column was filled with entries such as heart block (atherosclerosis), coma, carbuncle (a large abscess caused by a bacterial infection), carcinoma (cancer) of the pancreas, apoplexy (an old-time term for a stroke), myocardial infarction (a heart attack), cerebral embolism (again, stroke), and so on.

Diabetes's use of surrogates to deliver its death blow may help explain the public's apathy toward the disease—which in turn may help explain why the disease is spreading more like a virus. When the ADA held focus groups to gauge the public perception of the health threat posed by diabetes, on a scale of 1 to 10, people tended to assign 9s and 10s to cancer and heart disease but only 4s and 5s to diabetes. I'm reminded of a quote from the Kevin Spacey character in the movie *The Usual Suspects*: "The greatest trick the devil ever pulled was convincing the world he doesn't exist."

Your bloodstream is supposed to contain a teaspoon or so of glucose at any given moment. Tissues begin suffering damage when this small amount rises by even one-fourth. The simplest explanation of how higher-than-normal rates of glucose can contribute to the long-term complications of diabetes is that sugar gunks up the works. The higher the concentrations, the stickier the situation becomes. The linings of arteries and capillaries begin suffering damage. Free radicals run amok in both muscle and fat. High blood pressure, atherosclerosis, and diabetes likely aren't far behind.

If the most vexing aspect of diabetes is the number of different systems it attacks, the most promising aspect is that it's so plastic and modifiable. It's not like being told, *Okay, you just suffered a heart attack* or *There's a tumor in this part of your brain.* You can be diagnosed with type 2 diabetes and still reverse it, or at least keep it at bay for a long, long time. To do that, however, more attention needs to be paid to excessive insulin as a villain, and not just as a passive, supporting actor to high blood glucose. Many of the experts with whom I spoke said that diabetes should be thought of first and foremost as a disease of insulin malfunction, and secondarily as a disease of glucose deregulation.

"We now know that insulin resistance is a major factor in a variety of diseases, including PCOS, many forms of cancer, sleep apnea—I could go on and on," says Dr. Reaven. "The range of problems linked to it has grown over the past two decades."

BEFORE DIABETES ENTERED my life, what I knew about insulin came from being editor in chief of *Muscle & Fitness* magazine. And the lesson was a simple one: Insulin is incredibly powerful stuff.

Some hardcore bodybuilders find the intersection of training and insulin intoxicating. If a guy's doing three-a-days at Gold's Venice, eating sixteen egg whites and five chicken breasts for lunch, and taking enough anabolic steroids and human growth hormone to stock a Tijuana pharmacy, his lean tissue will appear to grow like time-lapsed photography. Amplifying growth into the realm of the extreme requires insulin, and a pro bodybuilder seldom settles for what his pancreas can produce by itself.

In the 1990s, bodybuilders figured out that they could inject insulin like a type 1 diabetic. But their objective wasn't survival; it was accumulating the sort of beef a prize steer displays at the county fair. Under this scenario, the influx of injected insulin and other growth factors sets off another damaging cascade, this time not in the sedentary person but in the lifter.

"Pairing insulin with human growth hormone and, more recently, insulinlike growth factor 1 has produced a spectrum of pathologies including kidney problems, vision problems, atherosclerosis, and heart-valve damage," says Jeff Feliciano, a former steroid chemist who came above ground as a sought-after formulator of high-performance dietary supplements. "Not the least of which is *unbridled* hypertension. Guys walking around with their blood pressure at 210 over 120, which just fries your kidneys."

The trend continues. When I interviewed several of the individuals who oversee the contest prep of the current crop of pro bodybuilders, they estimated that three-fourths of today's competitors have used insulin for physique enhancement at some point in their career.

For Arnold Schwarzenegger's generation, steroid use often led to cardiovascular problems later in life, including heart valve damage. But the guys I covered for *Muscle & Fitness* in the late 1990s and early 2000s—relatively young men who routinely used insulin to help blast their anabolic cocktails into muscle cells—tended to suffer kidney disease *first*, in their mid-to-late thirties, even before heart disease had become lethal. Off the top of my head, I can name five top bodybuilders of that era—guys I interviewed for the magazine—who were hooked up to a dialysis machine before celebrating their fortieth birthday.

This litany resembles the more protracted damage wrought by diabetes upon the sedentary and often overweight. Both the hardcore and inactive groups offer a lesson: Insulin is a powerful sword, complete with two very sharp edges. Many competitive bodybuilders embrace insulin as a shortcut to a freaky-huge, ripped physique, where conversely many diabetics abuse it in lieu of leading a healthier lifestyle. The trick is to make this powerful hormone work for rather than against you.

"Normally, insulin has some fairly positive effects on the body, such as being an anti-inflammatory," says Volek. "But if you're insulin resistant, chronically high insulin levels have the opposite effect. They actually promote inflammation and cardiovascular problems. That's not generally appreciated yet; what is well accepted is that high glucose will cause problems over time. So the primary target in diabetes treatment has been aggressive glucose lowering. Doctors will pump you full of insulin to keep the glucose down and not really worry about the long-term effects of the insulin."

The route to a diabetic death is littered with amputations, organ failures, and heartbreak, literal and figurative. You don't burn out from diabetes; you rust away. When I first saw my father after being out of touch with him for twenty years, I immediately understood what Dr. Barnett meant when he referred to diabetes as "metabolic leprosy." Consider the following effects of high blood glucose levels, of the extra insulin secreted to lower it, or of both:

• Cancer, as it turns out, has a sweet tooth. Recent research shows that the consumption of high amounts of sugar and refined grains boosts the odds for cancers of the esophagus, kidneys, and pancreas. Excessive insulin, produced internally in response to high glucose, appears to raise your risk of being diagnosed with a number of cancers, including breast and liver. "The link between obesity and cancer may not reflect obesity itself so much as insulin levels being high," says Stanford's Dr. Reaven. "The obese are likely to be insulin resistant and therefore produce too much of the hormone."

Cancer risk also appears to rise, and dramatically, among type 2 diabetics undergoing prolonged insulin therapy. One study found that each additional year of insulin therapy raised the risk of colorectal cancer by 20 percent.

On a recent flight I took, Northwest Airlines was promoting Breast Cancer Awareness month. Flight attendants dressed in commemorative pink outfits strode the aisles offering Minute Maid pink lemonade—40 grams of sugar per twelve ounces—for $2, with proceeds earmarked for the Breast Cancer Research Foundation. Undoubtedly the airline and its employees mean well. But one of the best ways to fight breast cancer may be to stop drinking concentrated forms of sugar. The fact that some whiz in marketing realized that Breast Cancer Awareness month and pink lemonade have matching colors doesn't change that reality.

• High blood sugar can sour your mood. In a recent study, researchers found that people who drink two and a half cans of sugary soda daily are three times more likely to be depressed and anxious than those drinking less pop. What's more, the depressed have a heightened risk for type 2 diabetes. The reverse also holds true: Diabetics are twice as likely as others to suffer depression.

• Diabetes can literally drive you crazy. High glucose levels provide fertile soil for plaque-forming proteins that can wreck brain neurons, increasing the odds of dementia, and then speeding it up once it begins. Particularly vulnerable is the region of the brain where learning occurs and memories are stored. Some researchers with whom I spoke believe that Alzheimer's disease may be a sort of "type 3" diabetes, a provocative but as yet unproven theory.

• High blood glucose levels can break your heart. When researchers study large populations, elevated blood sugar levels correlate with a greatly increased risk of heart disease, the number one killer of Americans. Diabetics are more than twice as likely as nondiabetics to suffer a heart attack. In fact, a diabetic has the same heart attack odds as a nondiabetic who's already had one.

• The prospect of having a stroke hangs over the head of everyone with diabetes. Even the young are more susceptible to these brain attacks once type 2 diabetes takes hold. Diabetic stroke survivors also tend to face more-crippling aftereffects than nondiabetics do. The climb back up from this devastating health setback will likely be rockier.

Thank high blood pressure for much of the increased stroke risk among diabetics. You want your heart's rhythmic *ba-boom*—and the resulting force of blood against the arterial walls—to be easy, not difficult. Higher-than-normal spells trouble ahead. The San Antonio Heart Study concluded that high insulin levels, both fasting and postmeal, predict hypertension in the normal-weight and overweight alike. The hormonal response to high blood sugar that crashes is like having three or four panic attacks a day. That'll jack up anyone's blood pressure.

• Your joints might ache and creak prematurely, too. A study published in the *Scandinavian Journal of Rheumatology* linked insulin resistance with rheumatoid arthritis. Arthritic inflammation has been associated not only with decreased insulin sensitivity but also with other metabolic syndrome components such as low HDL. The connection works both ways: Rheumatoid arthritis sufferers are more likely than others to become diabetic.

- The kidney disease rate is 22 percent higher among diabetic men than among all men, and diabetes is the leading cause of irreversible kidney disease requiring dialysis or kidney transplantation. The second-leading cause of end-stage kidney disease is hypertension, and the same thing that causes diabetes often causes that: insulin resistance. See how this is all connected? Our nation has roughly 300,000 people whose survival depends on dialysis.

- Diabetes skyrockets the risk of developing nonalcoholic fatty liver disease, as extra triglycerides produced from carbs overrun the organ. Most people with this condition lack obvious signs or symptoms and can be blindsided by cirrhosis or liver failure. Diabetes complications such as obesity and high LDL cholesterol also raise the odds of liver disease. One study I read suggested that diabetes may double the risk of chronic liver disease and liver cancer.

- If passing on jelly doughnuts seems difficult, imagine living without eyesight. In fact, nothing causes more new cases of blindness among twenty- to seventy-four-year-olds than diabetes. Say good-bye to twenty-twenty vision, since diabetics have a fifty-fifty chance of experiencing damage to the tiny blood vessels in the back of the eye. Blockages keep blood from flowing where it needs to go, and fluid leaks into places it shouldn't, turning the human eyeball into an ugly mess of scar tissue. Each year, twelve thousand to twenty-four thousand people lose their sight because of this process, called diabetic retinopathy. Diabetics are also at higher risk for cataracts and glaucoma.

- At least you'll still have your hearing, right? A recent study in *Annals of Internal Medicine* revealed that diabetics are more than twice as likely as nondiabetics to lose at least some hearing. The researchers speculated that over time, the tiny blood vessels in the cochlea might become damaged like the ones in the retina.

- Along the way, your teeth will rot. In part because too-high blood glucose damages the salivary glands, diabetes raises the risk for gum infections. Researchers at Columbia University recently established that the reverse is true as well: Those with periodontal disease have a greater risk of later becoming diabetic. They speculated that gum disease might somehow trigger diabetes, but I'm guessing that the same sugary diet causing the gum disease led to diabetes as well.

• It doesn't take much to interfere with the complex hydraulic system of blood vessels and nerves needed to hoist and maintain an erection, and you'd be hard-pressed to find a more common culprit than high blood sugar. Diabetes accounts for 30 percent of all U.S. erectile dysfunction cases. This problem will strike 35 to 50 percent of diabetic men, and onset typically occurs ten to fifteen years earlier in diabetics than in nondiabetics. Diabetes damages small blood vessels first. So, guys, first your penis goes, then your heart and brain follow suit. Do I have your attention yet?

Women aren't spared when it comes to the bedroom, either. Diabetes tends to diminish their sex drive, promote vaginal dryness, and short-circuit their orgasms.

• Women with diabetes have a narrower fertility window than nondiabetic women. They'll typically begin menstruating later and then enter menopause earlier than nondiabetic women. Many women with type 2 diabetes also have PCOS, which can result from excessive insulin production. They often have increased difficulty conceiving.

• Over time, diabetics often develop nerve damage, usually starting in the feet. Some diabetics wouldn't feel a flame there, let alone an infection abrew. Even the stomach's nerves are prone to a loss of sensation, and as a result up to half of those with long-standing diabetes experience delayed stomach emptying. A diabetic who takes insulin after a meal, only to have that meal sit in their stomach, is prone to hypoglycemia. Once controlling your blood sugar requires drugs, you're not really in control of anything anymore.

• Diabetes sows its evil seeds and then forces those who normally restore our bodies to cut them apart instead. In the public's mind, "diabetic" and "amputee" are nearly synonymous. No wonder: The disease is responsible for the loss of about 84,000 limbs every year. Five out of every thousand diabetics will experience an amputation, and more than 60 percent of nontrauma lower-limb amputations occur in people with diabetes. The 1.9 million U.S. amputees represent three-quarters of a million more than there were ten years ago. Prosthetics sales have nearly doubled, to $600 million, since 1996.

• Researchers have found that diabetes damages the DNA in a man's sperm. "This damage has a serious and detrimental effect on the ability of an embryo produced from the sperm to grow, implant, and then survive pregnancy," says Con Mallidis, Ph.D., head of andrology at the Centre for Reproductive Medicine and Andrology at the University of Münster in Germany. As yet no evidence connects this DNA-damaged sperm with increased birth defects if a child is conceived. According to Mallidis, however, a connection has been suggested between this sperm damage and the onset of some childhood illnesses, including cancers.

• Blood sugar gyrations can lead to insomnia and other sleep disorders. When blood sugar crashes, your body detects the change and sets off an internal alarm clock: *Hey, you! Get up! You need food!* What's more, type 2 diabetes and sleep apnea seem to keep company in ways that aren't yet well understood. Sleep interruptions appear to increase the formation of blood clots, a predictor of heart disease.

WHICH BRINGS US back to the biggest killer of them all: heart disease. It kills three-fourths of all diabetics. Diabetes is a metabolic disease *and* a vascular disease, so coronary disease is implicit. Diabetes and heart disease often share a root cause: insulin resistance. Its signature effects—hyperglycemia, high triglycerides, low HDL, and hypertension—are leading risk factors for type 2 diabetes and heart disease alike.

"I was trained that if you walked in and saw a forty-seven-year-old diabetic who'd been on insulin for twenty-five years, and he was in for gall bladder surgery, you'd work him up as if he were seventy-two years old," says Dr. Barnett. "Because he may have a coronary during this gall bladder surgery. He may be forty-seven, but you should prepare him as if he were his father!"

Heart disease, and not type 2 diabetes, has been the serial killer in my paternal lineage. My father's mother, Ada, was one of seven children born to Hugh and Martha Gibson. In their prime, the siblings shared a casual elegance; in old, yellowing photos they are tall, trim, stylish, and remind me of F. Scott Fitzgerald characters. The heart inside every single one of them stopped beating prematurely, a fate that has befallen many of their children—my paternal aunts and uncles. The keeper of much of this family history, my father's brother and my godfather, Hughie O'Connell, underwent a quintuple bypass three months after running a marathon at age fifty-nine.

Many of these individuals' descendants never knew if their parents were prediabetic or diabetic. But if many people alive today don't know that their blood sugar has gone berserk, how about someone born in, say, 1918? What chance did he or she have? Even now, diabetes is often diagnosed only after someone survives a heart attack.

Diabetes and prediabetes impair the functioning of the endothelium, stiffen formerly relaxed arteries, inflame tissues throughout the cardio-vascular system, and can lead to a dangerous condition known as left ventricular diastolic dysfunction, in which the heart cannot properly fill with blood. "At the time of their diabetes diagnosis, up to 25 percent of patients will have a positive exercise stress test," says Kerry J. Stewart, Ed.D., director of clinical and research exercise physiology at Johns Hopkins University School of Medicine. A cardiac stress test subjects a patient to exercise on a treadmill and then measures electrical activity in the heart. A positive result means trouble. Patients with diabetes should be treated as though they have heart disease, according to Stewart.

Heart disease can occur in the absence of blood sugar problems and major insulin resistance, too. LDL cholesterol, for example, contributes to atherosclerosis but doesn't fit snugly under metabolic syndrome's umbrella. When insulin resistance is addressed, LDL doesn't automatically right itself the way HDL, triglycerides, blood pressure, and blood glucose tend to do. As Dr. Reaven notes, if you have insulin resistance *and* a genetic predisposition to high numbers of small-size LDL particles, you're on a collision course with heart disease. That would include me and, I'm sure, many of my relatives, those living, and those prematurely dead. I've attempted evasive action.

I have a theory that the heart attacks that killed my relatives may have more to do with my father's and my diabetic issues than one might assume—and that this may be repeated in families across America. We feast on carb-dense foods that send our blood sugars soaring and crashing all day long, and the harder we crash, the stronger the pick-me-ups. Drinking a cup of coffee (90 to 150 milligrams of caffeine) with a tablespoon of sugar (12.6 grams' worth) seems almost quaint at this point. For more caffeine, people reach for drinks such as Shock Coffee Triple Latte, Spike Shotgun, and Wired, which contain two or three times that amount. For more sugar, they can opt for Hype (67.5 grams per can), Minute Maid Cranberry Grape (72.2 grams in a 15.2-ounce bottle), and Sunkist Orange Soda (52 grams per can). Most of these types of drinks combine both stimulants: caffeine and some version of sugar. The best seller in the category is Red Bull. Worldwide, people consume about four billion cans a year.

It's well documented that blood sugar spikes and crashes damage the inner walls of our arteries. A team of Italian researchers recently identified a mechanism by which blood sugar swings among even *nondiabetics* leads to high blood pressure and heart disease. They attempted to correlate two variables on a hunch. The first was blood sugar variability— how much it moves, regardless of whether the actual levels were high, low, or normal. If you follow the stock market, this calculation is like the CBOE Volatility Index, as opposed to the S&P 500. The second variable was the performance of the internal walls of blood vessels, which are composed of endothelial cells.

The researchers stratified sixty subjects into three groups—normal, nondiabetic with metabolic syndrome, and diabetic—and had them wear continuous glucose monitors for two days. They didn't average the several thousand blood sugar readings that were generated, which would be the net effect of an A1C test. Instead they calculated standard deviations from the mean. At the same time, they took highly sensitive measurements of working arteries. Did they relax, like they should in response to blood flow? Or did they stiffen, as in hardening of the arteries? A poor score on the test they used correlates with cardiovascular complications.

The correlation in this experiment was strong, and alarming: the

greater the fluctuations, the more damage, regardless of the actual glucose amounts. "These blood sugar fluctuations, even among those who
are not yet diabetic, are toxic for the endothelium," said the lead researcher, Silvio Buscemi, M.D., Ph.D., when I met him standing in
front of his poster at the ADA conference. He works at the University
of Palermo in Italy as a researcher and professor specializing in diabetes
and clinical nutrition, and as an internist at the university's hospital.

What's more, the second group, those with only metabolic syndrome,
not (yet) diabetes, had high variability, the kind that causes heart
disease—even though many of them had normal fasting glucose scores
and A1Cs. As I mentioned, though hailed for their predictive power by
the diabetes establishment, these two tests are often lagging indicators.
In fact people with relatively low blood sugar but high variability had
the same impaired endothelial function as people with high blood
sugar and low variability.

Dr. Buscemi believes that we're looking at only part of the picture
right now, with deadly consequences. "Fasting plasma glucose tells us
something," he says. "Postmeal glucose, something else; A1C, something
else. Glycemic variability is another marker, one that we think accounts
for a percentage of the explained risk of cardiovascular disease. Integrating the data would provide a better explanation."

The diabetic process is already happening before our fasting blood
sugar reading even enters the red zone. The first sign of trouble doctors
identify isn't a particularly reliable measure of glucose tolerance. Before
the fasting number rises to a level that's red-flagged by standard tests,
postmeal blood sugar spikes, during which the most serious damage occurs, have been occurring for months or years. A test exists that reveals
these two-hour spikes—it's the one that challenges the metabolic system with a sugary drink. Yet people are seldom asked to take it. Many
doctors and patients think administering this test is a hassle, although
surely it's less of a hassle than dealing with heart attacks, amputations,
and dialysis later.

Instead we wait until the damage is so obvious that we're dialing 911,
and then we expect someone to pull out a medical toolbox, filled with

arterial stents and prescriptions and other instruments, and "fix" a problem that could have been prevented, or at least delayed.

Many of the folks who suddenly slump at their desks or never wake up from a night's sleep in their forties or fifties were probably well on their way to type 2 diabetes. They just suffered a fatal heart attack first.

It was, in most cases, preventable.

6

THE GRAVE CONSEQUENCE
OF DENIAL

'm transfixed by the view of snow-frosted mountain peaks soaring before me. Two nights earlier, their outlines and shadows had loomed courtesy of the sort of full moon drawn in a children's book. I was behind the wheel of a rented Ford Escape near midnight, having been on the road since morning, driving north from Vancouver before hanging a left at Prince George and heading due west toward the ocean. Dead tired. In an attempt to stay awake, I had rolled down the windows and blared Jimmy Buffett's Radio Margaritaville on Sirius for the last leg of my drive. I wasn't keen on plowing into a wayward moose at eighty-five miles an hour. I'd already seen a wild horse galloping down the highway in my headlights.

Daylight makes those peaks seem farther away, and majestic rather than ominous. I'm on the Bulkley River in northern British Columbia with three other men. We're strangers but all in the same boat, touched in some way by diabetes. Also on board is Dr. Wortman, here on behalf of the First Nations and Inuit Health Branch of Health Canada; he's prediabetic and something of a renegade in his approach to treating the disease. Bob Haslett, an avid outdoorsman who spent decades working as a lineman for British Columbia's largest telephone company before retiring, has a wife named Doreen with type 1 diabetes. Our guide for the day is Wayne Gray, owner of a landscaping and construction company. His wife, Sarah, is a professor researching diabetes and obesity at the University of Northern British Columbia.

The biggest surprise I experienced while researching this book is that I haven't met one person who hasn't been touched in some way by this sugar scourge. Even if the person I'm talking to doesn't have the disease or the inklings of it, there's sure to be a wife or husband, brother or sister, parent or grandparent, aunt or uncle, boss, coworker, or friend who does. The same might be said of cancer, but diabetes seems even more ingrained in our society. After all, with cancer you either survive it, or it kills you, whereas type 2 diabetes doesn't go away, at least not with the prevailing treatments. For many it's a curse to be accepted rather than an adversary to be challenged or rebuffed. All too often, however, fatalism pervades not only patients but also doctors and health organizations.

The type 2 diabetes crisis is spreading globally as fast as Internet access and cell phone coverage. Technology itself may be part of the problem: It's driving the desire for all things Western, including the manufactured diet and leisurely lifestyle that are quietly killing Americans. The IDF has periodically published its diabetes "atlas," and in the 2000 inaugural edition, India and China were estimated to have thirty-three million and twenty-three million diabetics, respectively. In the most recent edition, from October 2009, India now has fifty-one million diabetics, twice the number of diabetics in the United States. China, with forty-three million, was second. (Type 2 diabetes seems to strike Indians at least ten to fifteen years earlier than it does other nationalities.) According to IDF's report, which was based on the best available data at the time, India and China have a slightly lower percentage of the population with diabetes than the United States. They also have many more people, and hence more total diabetics.

But there may be even more than we thought, and it goes back to the blood glucose testing limitations and deficiencies I discussed earlier. In

March 2010, the *New England Journal of Medicine* published study findings based on a "nationally representative sample" of 46,239 Chinese adults, who were all given a glucose tolerance test. The percentage rates for both diabetes and prediabetes were twofold higher than the IDF figures. So that forty-three million number for Chinese diabetics? Make that ninety-two million, a conclusion that the IDF accepted in a press release. The same testing suggests 148 million prediabetics. Whereas a quarter of all U.S. diabetics are in the dark about their dysfunctional glucose metabolism, 60 percent of the Chinese are.

Solve the diabetes pandemic? We haven't even begun to quantify the problem.

The disease is growing faster still in the Middle East. Thirty to 35 percent of the population of Saudi Arabia is now diabetic. Qatar, Bahrain, United Emirates—all these countries and more are in the midst of a collective blood sugar meltdown. What's happening is that Westernization and economic development are accelerating particularly fast in oil-producing nations. The result has been less physical activity, more calories, more obesity, and more smoking—a recipe for type 2 diabetes.

Yet the world's aboriginal populations, including our own Native American populations, are suffering the gravest consequences. "We don't know of any indigenous population that is diabetes-free once they're Coca-Cola–nized," says Dr. Zimmet, of the Baker IDI Heart and Diabetes Institute.

To conduct his seminal field research on native populations and type 2 diabetes, Dr. Zimmet traveled to Nauru, a lush dot in the central Pacific. Before World War II brought the native population into contact with Westerners—soldiers, in this case—the island was a tropical paradise unblemished by type 2 diabetes. Now it seems more like hell on Earth. More than one-third of the adults in Nauru have the disease, not to mention similar rates of kidney failure, blindness, and other diabetes complications.

The same fate has befallen those members of Australia's indigenous population who've migrated to urban centers and begun eating like the locals. "They have the highest rates of kidney failure and dialysis in the world," says Dr. Zimmet. Then there are the people of Tonga, where 84 percent of the men and 93 percent of the women are overweight or obese. These numbers are climbing, too. Populations have been starved into extinction before, but the Tongans may become the first group in human history to eat its way off the planet.

This isn't merely a tropical tragedy. The four of us are afloat in this boat because, the day before, the Smithers chapter of the Canadian Diabetes Association (CDA) had hosted its first diabetes expo in four years. Part of the Gitxsan First Nation, Smithers lies west of Prince George and east of Prince Rupert on the Yellowhead Highway. This gathering bore scant resemblance to the ADA's diabetes extravaganza in New Orleans. Here the venue was the Della Herman Theatre, inside Smithers Senior Secondary School. But instead of Canadian teens hamming up *The Pirates of Penzance*, diabetes experts, Dr. Wortman among them, were offering sober presentations. Outside the auditorium were several sexy female drug reps who had been flown in to adorn simple booths. Some things don't change from one diabetes conference to the next. Lunch was served in what I'm guessing is the school's cafeteria.

A day later, I find myself holding a rod and reel for the first time since high school. Trolling a wide, muscular river takes skill and energy; this is no lazy man's Sunday afternoon. Wading waist high, I step onto rocks along the bottom, a balancing act that reminds me of those $250-an-hour functional workouts championed by Hollywood trainers. I rotate at the waist in my rubber wading pants to launch a cast toward the spot where Wayne has assured me the prized steelhead trout lie waiting and hungry. I fling my line, but my right foot shoots off a mossy rock. Every muscle in my core clenches for balance, but I lose control and splash sideways, the rod flying from my hand. Frigid water pours into the thigh-high rubber pants.

"You got a little closer to the fish than you had wanted, eh?" says one of my shipmates for the day, as the other two roar with laughter. I've never been an outdoorsman, but apparently guys are supposed to know how to do this. Whatever. I have bigger fish to fry on this trip: type 2 diabetes and its devastating consequences.

We're fishing with modern-day gear, but the indigenous inhabitants once used only spears and nets to catch the salmon, steelhead, and

other fish forging up rivers like this one in order to spawn. With sustenance at stake, a fisherman could burn a ton of calories hanging over a
bank and using a dip net to pull up fifty- and sixty-pound spring salmon.
The meal these fish provided would offer more than 20 grams of protein
and a few grams of healthy fat. Adding carbs from a handful of wild
vegetables or berries creates a perfect meal for maintaining metabolic
health. Their weight-loss regimen would beat the heck out of anything
being hawked on infomercials. But they didn't need to lose weight.

In the Stone Age, whole communities would paddle for days or
weeks in search of a certain fish. Smelt, they're called, and they contain
a predominantly monounsaturated fat, called oolichan grease, that could
be harvested in temporary camps along the shore, stored for long periods, and used as needed, even as currency. This marine fat might have
accounted for half the energy consumption of some of the First Nations' distant forebearers. "Centuries ago, these people figured out that
among the array of fats available in their surroundings, the oil from this
little fish was worth all that effort to extract and consume because it
was the most appropriate fat to eat," says Dr. Wortman.

In addition to salmon and steelhead, other staples of the traditional
aboriginal diet included dozens of different meats (moose, bear, porcu-
pine, caribou, elk, sheep), more seafood (cod, whitefish, snapper, sea
urchin, octopus), birds (quail, pheasant, grouse, partridge), and eggs
(herring, salmon, seagull, goose, duck), according to a brochure I'm
handed at the Canadian diabetes conference. The First Nations peoples
also munched on a variety of berries and vegetables. The carbs these
contain aren't the starchy and sugary kinds. Of all the food groups
listed on the brochure, the category with the fewest entries is "bread
and cereals" (rice, rice root, Indian bread, and cooked cereal). Even the
list of barks (cedar, inner), fats (moose), and other greases (bear, deer,
seal) is longer.

As in rural Mississippi, things have changed here. Most of the an-
glers are like the well-heeled Italian sport fishers we encountered at a
local diner, or Dick Cheney types in search of trophy catches. (I was
told that, two weeks after I left, the former vice president, surrounded
by bodyguards, did indeed stop at the Bulkley to do some fishing.) But

the First Nations residents who actually live here are more likely to use their government assistance checks to purchase noodles and other cheap, convenient carbs. The dichotomy I saw in Mississippi—lush farmland on the one hand, locals living on junk food on the other—exists in coastal B.C. as well. Here, though, rivers are the bountiful food source.

The day before the diabetes conference, I joined Dr. Wortman as he made the rounds of several smaller towns to the east and west of Smithers. At a small presentation the doctor gave in Hazelton at a thirty-bed hospital operated by the United Church of Canada, a Gitxsan chief named Brian Williams, from the village of Kispiox, listened intently before responding: "You talk about our traditional foods such as seafood, and, yes, we eat a lot of fish and so on, but boredom sets in. Someone eating fish every day watches the next person eat fries, burgers, chicken chow mein at all these Chinese restaurants around here. How do you go about convincing them to resist eating that stuff?"

ECHOING THE NAURU experience, type 2 diabetes wasn't even detected in Canada's aboriginals fifty years ago. Today researchers, policy makers, and the aboriginal communities themselves all speak of the type 2 diabetes epidemic, a phrase repeated so often that it's now shopworn rather than shocking. A study done in Manitoba, another Canadian province, projected that for the two decades ending in 2016, diabetes will have been responsible for "a tenfold increase in the rate of cardiovascular disease; a fivefold increase in strokes; ten times as many dialysis starts; ten times the rate of lower extremity amputations; and five times the rate of blindness among aboriginal peoples." These populations are being taken apart, literally and figuratively.

At the national level in Canada, no one in a position of authority seems to know what to do. The concern is no doubt genuine, and bureaucracies do what bureaucracies do: Cut the occasional check, hold conferences, make promises, and wring their hands. But nothing is working. "This disaster is happening in slow motion," says Dr. Wortman. "It's not like an earthquake hit these people. What's the headline to galvanize action? It's out of sight, out of mind."

Dr. Wortman has few allies, and not by choice. He wants to win converts who can actually help him influence diabetes policy at the national level. So he's delighted when we're joined for dinner one evening by Brian Rodrigues, Ph.D., professor at the University of British Columbia. The professor happens to sit on the board of directors of the Canadian Diabetes Association.

Dr. Rodrigues looks Indian to me but has a Portuguese surname, and I struggle to place his accent. As it turns out, he's from Goa, a state along India's coast that was first conquered by the Portuguese. His obsession with fishing is immediately apparent, and I sense that a promised excursion has lured him to this remote conference. Talk of steelhead fill the initial banter, with Rodrigues speaking in rapid-fire bursts punctuated by high-pitched laughter. He's a nerd, but he's an engaging and charismatic nerd, and very sharp.

The conversation segues to the subject of diabetes, with Dr. Wortman hitting his low-carb talking points. Earlier I'd heard him lecture other doctors, nurses, diabetes educators, and nutritionists. He's smart, well informed, and smooth talking; listeners tend to be persuaded or threatened, but I hadn't seen him challenged yet. I enjoy listening to him pitch his theories to an academician who is at least his intellectual peer. Both men acquit themselves admirably during our dinner discussion, and I'm the beneficiary.

Rodrigues teaches in the pharmaceutical sciences, so I'm pleasantly surprised when he agrees about the necessity of lifestyle medicine leading the way in diabetes prevention and care. He doesn't say so, but I sense that he isn't swayed by Wortman's low-carb pitch. He seems more receptive to my two cents on the power of exercise.

"Any dessert for you tonight?" asks the waitress. "We have a homemade chocolate cheesecake that just came out of the oven tonight."

"That's *very* tempting, but I'm resisting," says Dr. Wortman.

"You have a stronger willpower than I do," says the waitress.

Over coffee, my dinner mates talk about finding a drug for her dilemma, one that would override that most basic of human impulses: hunger. "Will we ever be able to develop a pill [for that]?" asks Rodrigues rhetorically. "I doubt it. They do all these 'knockout' studies, where they knock this out and knock that out." He's referring to decommissioning certain genes in experimental mice, so that the function of those genes can be inferred by comparing them to mice with those genes intact. "But so many things are compensating [for the knocked-out sequence]. There's so much redundancy in the system. So many of the new diabetes drug ideas come from genetic engineering, but then they can't duplicate it in humans."

SPEAKING OF HUNGER and diabetes, at the conference I also picked up a pamphlet titled *Eating Well with Canada's Food Guide*, produced by Health Canada. (In Canada, the main health organization, rather than the agriculture department, develops the food guidelines.) Unlike the old USDA pyramid, this arrangement prioritizes foods from top to bottom. Along the upper row lie vegetables and fruit (seven servings a day), including sugary fruits such as bananas and fruit juice. Below that are grain products (seven servings a day). Then come milk and alternatives, such as yogurt (three servings). The brochure encourages diabetics to eat plentifully from the food groups that made them diabetic in the first place.

Along the bottom lie meat and alternatives (three servings), which include foods that would have fit with the traditional diet. Even there, readers are encouraged to swap tofu for meat if possible. I've interviewed Dr. Wortman several times over meals during the weekend, and I can't help but notice that this diabetes expert from Health Canada wouldn't touch most of what's on his employer's recommended list with a ten-foot pole.

The vexing question is: Why does the type 2 diabetes problem seem even worse here than it does among nonindigenous Canadians? This anthropology lesson is unfolding all across the planet: Every time a native population forsakes homegrown food for manufactured food, and becomes sedentary rather than active, diabetes rears its head, as if on cue. Aboriginal populations seem to have the very lowest threshold for carbohydrates, making them especially vulnerable to type 2 diabetes. Even modest weight gain brings out a genetic predisposition that was previously overcome by physical activity of the sort needed to survive centuries and millennia ago.

"Aboriginals might as well have been ripped right out of the Stone Age," says RMIT University's Mann. "They have only three, four generations at most separating them from the time when their ancestors hunted and foraged for food that was exceptionally healthy. That's given them no time for genetic adaptation to the Western food they're suddenly consuming instead of the diet that was perfectly suited for their bodies: lean meat from wild animals, fish, and plants."

These people also tend to be inherently insulin resistant. As strange as it sounds today, some degree of insulin resistance once offered a survival advantage. Researchers have found that three-quarters of hunter-gatherer societies worldwide ate other animals rather than plants for their sustenance. Those diets tended to include lots of protein and variable amounts of fat but few carbs. So bodies that burned a ton of calories clung to those carbs as if life depended on it—which it did. They clung by becoming a little insulin resistant.

Europeans, in contrast, have been exposed to agriculture for ten thousand years. At least some of that natural insulin resistance has been bred out of populations. The average European or North American has nowhere near the insulin resistance of an aboriginal.

"We've still not adapted to a carbohydrate-rich diet, but we're farther along the pathway than hunter-gatherer groups," says Mann. "That's why when you place Australian aboriginals and the Pima Indians on a Western diet, their rate of type 2 diabetes approaches 100 percent by the time they reach their forties. Virtually every aboriginal over fifty would have type 2 diabetes, with a life expectancy of another ten years, maybe. A massive disaster is unfolding among these native populations."

The Pima Indians, whose reservation lies south of Phoenix, are often used as a case study of what happens when aboriginal populations adopt a modern, fast-food lifestyle. The rates of type 2 diabetes and obesity have skyrocketed on the reservation. But the story is much different south of the Mexican border, among tribes forming part of the same ethnic group and sharing great genetic similarity with the Pima. These groups still follow their traditional diets, and their rates of obesity and diabetes remain low. Granted, much of the traditional fare in that part of the world consists of plant foods, which tend to be high in carbs, but they're eaten in an unrefined form. They're high in fiber. They're digested slowly as a result. What's more, these societies remain agrarian. Working the soil combines cardio and resistance training. Their energy intake and expenditure maintain a healthy equilibrium as a result.

When the traditional-to-Western dietary change is reversed in studies, the disease vanishes. "As unhealthy and fat and diabetic as the aboriginal subjects are, they become very healthy when they're put back on a hunter-gatherer-type diet," says Mann. "They lose weight, their blood glucose regulation improves, and their cardiovascular risk factors decrease."

Dr. Wortman participated in a similar study. A hundred or so Namgis First Nation residents of Alert Bay, Canada, were placed on today's version of the ancestral diet—Atkins. Salmon and halibut fit the bill for the study as they did in the distant past, but other traditional foods, such as seaweed and sea urchin, were replaced by market foods. Chicken and beef could stand in for caribou and moose. The experiment was to be filmed. Challenges ranged from native mistrust of white men in lab coats to the procarb, antifat philosophies of the Canadian health establishment. Yet another risk: Dr. Wortman, the low-carb guru, ending up with egg on his face, beloved yolks and all. "I made it clear to Jay that if we followed subjects who failed on the diet, that's what would end up in the documentary," said Mary Bissell, who directed *My Big Fat Diet* for the Canadian Broadcasting Corporation. "He took a big risk in having me observe this experiment."

None of which fazed Dr. Wortman, who has the sort of icy blue gaze and brushlike silver hair that normally earns a character actor a black turtleneck, a twitching eyebrow, and a detonator in a Jerry Bruckheimer movie. But he's a very nice, down-to-earth fellow. Still, the occasional convergence of devilish glare and bemused expression betrays a contrarian's bent that runs deep.

Conducted over a year among the Namgis, the Alert Bay pilot study produced noteworthy improvements in glucose control, waist-to-hip measures, cholesterol, triglycerides, and blood pressure. All were achieved with no calorie restriction, only different food choices. The documentary runs occasionally on national television in Canada, making Dr. Wortman a quasi-celebrity at these small diabetes gatherings. My sense is that he doesn't mind the attention.

Undoubtedly part of the experiment's success owed to peer pressure. "Group support is essential," says nutrition expert Jonny Bowden, who first directed me to the documentary. "Even Weight Watchers is one of these weird mergers of horrible nutritional advice with advanced social technique. The details change, but every twelve-step group in the world reproduces some form of the support group. That's what makes them work." In Alert Bay, however, the diet and social engineering worked in concert for a change.

Mann found exactly the same results in Australia that Dr. Wortman did in Alert Bay. "No matter how much we told the young men in our studies to eat of all these more-natural, traditional foods, they would lose weight, because natural foods have a lot of protein and a lower energy density," he says. "They couldn't help but lose weight. Many other health parameters having to do with heart disease, such as unhealthy cholesterol and triglycerides, also went down. That's not so important yet for these young boys, but if those parameters dropped for them, imagine what it would do to middle-age adults with high cholesterol and triglycerides. We've replicated the study in them, and the dietary switch does lower those markers."

EVEN WITHIN INDUSTRIALIZED countries, type 2 diabetes appears to do its own form of racial profiling. The 26.8 million diabetics in the United States represent 8.7 percent of the U.S. population. Yet this percentage is even higher among minority populations such as Alaska natives, African Americans, and Hispanics, which includes Puerto Ricans, Mexican Americans, and Cubans. Two groups falling below the mean are Asian Americans (7.5 percent) and whites (6.6 percent). Asians don't seem to need as much excess weight as Caucasians for the disease to take hold. They become sicker at lower BMIs, further proof that body weight and type 2 diabetes aren't always correlated.

Young Hispanics have the greatest lifetime risk of developing diabetes, followed by their African American counterparts. A Hispanic woman has a greater than 50 percent risk of developing diabetes in her lifetime. Yet, in general, men are slightly more likely than women to turn diabetic.

How tempting to blame it all on Mom and Dad. In fact, researchers around the world have identified thirty or so genes as having common variations that predispose people to type 2 diabetes. Jaakko Tuomilehto, M.D., Ph.D., professor of public health at the University of Helsinki and a member of the Diabetes Prevention Unit at the National Institute for Health and Welfare in Helsinki, Finland, makes a case for a prediabetic genotype, one that isn't tied to any specific glucose measures. Depending on how many of these diabetes-specific genes you possess, this theory goes, you may or may not be destined for diabetes.

This is a different way of looking at prediabetes, although I don't think it's a very compelling one. "Genetic variation alone clearly cannot explain the explosive increase in the incidence of non-insulin dependent [i.e., type 2] diabetes that occurs when underdeveloped populations adopt a Western lifestyle," wrote Stephen O'Rahilly, professor of metabolic medicine at the University of Cambridge.

At present, those thirty diabetes genes explain only 10 percent of overall susceptibility to diabetes. Ultimately, say the experts, genetics may account for up to 50 percent. That, to me, is cause for celebration—it leaves the other half to lifestyle, more than enough for you to kick type 2 diabetes's tail. Culture plays a role as well. In China, for example, memories of famine lead to the overfeeding of children. Another problem is that many Chinese don't like having their blood drawn for lab work.

Since type 2 diabetes is but one expression of metabolic syndrome, opposing camps have engaged in a vigorous nature-versus-nurture debate. One camp argues that obesity, diabetes, and heart disease share common characteristics, such as abnormal lipid levels, which result from matching lifestyle choices—say, eating unhealthy foods. Another group says that certain people experience elevations in blood sugar, LDL cholesterol, and blood pressure—followed by diabetes, heart disease, or both—because common genes heighten the risk for all of those health problems.

"We can't easily untangle the two factors [genetics and lifestyle] at this time, and I don't think there's a clear answer," Wake Forest University's Bowden told me. "It's a major research question: What do all of these things ultimately fit back to? Where are they connected?"

DR. WORTMAN WANTS to find out. He's the son of a Caucasian man who served as a Canadian Air Force pilot and a woman who is Métis, one of Canada's three aboriginal populations. They raised him in a village nestled on the banks of the Peace River in northern Alberta, where the temperature can dip to fifty below during the winter. He worked construction jobs in remote oil fields near the Northwest Territories for nearly a decade before changing his direction in life, entering medical school at age thirty-one.

Diabetes is a family heirloom: His mother and all eight of her siblings developed diabetes, heart disease, or both. Despite Dr. Wortman's medical degree and family history, diabetes snuck up on him, too. In 2002 he was tired, thirsty, peeing too much, and a little too heavy. But even he didn't connect the dots. It just so happens he had placed urinary dipsticks in the bathroom, thinking his son might be diabetic. The doc's son was okay, but one cold, rainy November day, he tested himself. His own blood sugar was sky high.

Knowing that carbs translate into glucose, Dr. Wortman sidestepped those foods while deciding what to do next. Meanwhile, his blood sugar fell back to normal. Which led him to wonder: Would carb cutting have a dramatic effect on the public-health catastrophe he saw among the aboriginals he'd visit as part of his job? He became convinced that it would, and this effort became his life's work.

Low-carb dieting is still a tough sell in these First Nations communities, even when the salesman has native blood and a big-time position with Health Canada. After finishing medical school at the University of Calgary and completing his family medicine residency at the University of British Columbia, Dr. Wortman became associate director of STD/HIV at the BC Centre for Disease Control in 1988. Prejudice, misunderstanding, and panic surrounded that epidemic in the late 1980s, but according to Dr. Wortman, his low-carb views elicit a more visceral negative reaction now than his HIV talks did back then. As the late anthropologist Margaret Mead once observed, "It is easier to change a man's religion [or sexual mores, in this case] than to change his diet."

When Dr. Wortman and I had first entered a small-town community center in South Hazelton that serves the Gitsegukla, a First Nations group, a young native woman wondered aloud if I was his bodyguard. "A few years ago, when [Dr. Wortman] came to give a presentation in Prince George, he was treated like the anti-Christ," explains Bill Goodacre. Our informal guide for much of the weekend, and a former local politician who serves as a member of CDA's national board, Goodacre is an instantly likable host who ambles about like a small bear, an effect accentuated by his mop of unkempt hair, scruffy beard, and chubby build. "But it's gotten better in the last two years, even," he adds, smiling at the doctor. "The word they use now is *controversy*."

"Instead of . . . ?" I ask.

"Well, they were using the word *heretic* before," he says, laughing.

I don't agree with everything Dr. Wortman has to say about diabetes. To me he, like many of Atkins's devotees, way underestimates the importance of exercise. Listening to him speak, I also find that Dr. Wortman gives short shrift to fiber's importance in glucose control and health in general—although, as he notes, nonstarchy vegetables, which he favors, do contain fiber. Fiber helps explain why the Pima could follow a traditional plant-based diet and be as unfamiliar with type 2 diabetes as the First Nations were on their protein-and-fat menu. No need to ship whale blubber to people who've lived in a desert for centuries, as long as they don't sit in air-conditioned rooms eating junk food and watching television all day.

When a low-carb diet isn't being asked to do everything by itself, when it's not the only joystick for glucose control, it doesn't have to be followed as relentlessly as these low-carb gurus insist. At least I don't think so. By syncing my diet with my workouts, I've found that I can control blood glucose to a degree that neither tool could alone. When Dr. Wortman and I attended a small gathering for the speakers, drug reps, and a few other guests held at a local church on Saturday night, moose lasagna was the featured item of a potluck. The doctor might as well be a surgeon, considering the dexterity with which he separated the moose meat from the pasta. I ate the dish as prepared. Hell, when would I ever have moose lasagna again? Anyway, I'd burn off those carbs with some wind sprints.

That said, on the fundamental issue of what diabetics should and shouldn't eat, I believe that Dr. Wortman's low-carb approach is right and that the majority's low-fat position is wrong.

One of Dr. Wortman's converts is Peter Newbery, M.D., who came to Hazelton as a young physician forty years ago. Back then, he says, he never encountered patients with type 2 diabetes; today his caseload reflects rates among nonnatives threefold Canada's national average. "Our communities will be facing enormous rising costs from people who are in renal failure, going blind, suffering heart attacks and strokes—some of which could be mitigated by what you're suggesting," said Dr. Newbery, nodding across the conference table to Dr. Wortman after his presentation at the United Church of Canada hospital. "I'm not saying it's simple, but it seems tremendously important to get this message across about how to avoid sugars and recognize the dangers they pose."

HOW TO FORTIFY cultures and nations against this modern-day plague? Ancestors of Dr. Wortman's may hold the key—not the Métis, but the Pennsylvania Dutch. Type 2 diabetes strikes the Amish, at least those living in Lancaster County, Pennsylvania, at one-half the frequency it hits the rest of the nation.

I wondered if the antidote to type 2 diabetes might lie in my own backyard, as I lived forty-five minutes east of Lancaster County. Making the drive one brisk January morning, I reached the crest of a long, rising stretch of two-lane country road when a fluorescent orange triangle attached to a black rectangle appeared through the mist. It was a horse and buggy, and I was approaching fast. Guiding one of those takes physical effort; fortunately, steering clear required only that I flick my steering wheel and hit the gas. Auto transport might be faster, but riding in a buggy burns more calories along the way.

My destination was the Amish Research Clinic, headquarters for a research team led by medical geneticist Alan R. Shuldiner, M.D. Nearly all of the Amish living in Lancaster County trace their lineage to two hundred individuals who were alive and procreating (a lot) in the eighteenth century. The Amish marry only their kind. Such exclusivity makes them perfect lab rats for researchers.

The clinic's story dates back to 1993, when Dr. Shuldiner was on the faculty at Johns Hopkins University. Looking to make his mark, he approached a colleague named Victor A. McKusick, M.D., who had pioneered the field of clinical medical genetics with his studies of the Amish in the 1950s and 1960s. Dr. McKusick made the necessary introductions.

Dr. Shuldiner and an Amish liaison went door to door, trying to convince Amish family members to sit for an in-home glucose-tolerance test. It wasn't as tough a sell as you might think. Because they don't believe in purchasing health insurance, the Amish prize free medical data, even if obtaining it means becoming a human guinea pig. They're not against advanced technology such as medical devices. They just don't want to be turning the knobs themselves.

The doctor also asked if he could extract DNA from their blood samples. He was ready when they said yes, having turned his car into a mobile laboratory, complete with portable gas-driven generator, a small centrifuge, and a chest of dry ice. After leaving a subject's house, Dr. Shuldiner would pop the hatchback of his Honda Accord and spin the blood, separate the serum, and freeze samples for the return trip to Baltimore. The DNA could be studied back at the lab.

In 1995, Dr. Shuldiner received funding from a drug maker and then NIH to open the clinic. In 1997, he and his team moved from Johns Hopkins to the University of Maryland School of Medicine in Baltimore.

Over nearly two decades, the research team has enrolled one-third of the entire Lancaster Amish population in various studies and performed nearly one billion genetic tests, looking for genes and chromosomal regions linked to diabetes and other metabolic syndrome problems. But their initial research, the Amish Family Diabetes Study, remains their masterpiece. Rather than finding any hardwired protection against type 2 diabetes, the researchers have found the same genetic variations that raise risk for the disease everywhere, and possibly some additional high-risk genes. "The Amish carry at least the same genetic burden for type 2 diabetes as the aboriginal groups," says Dr. Shuldiner, now head of University of Maryland School of Medicine's division of endocrinology, diabetes, and nutrition.

What's more, their diet is kind of a disaster, high in fat, carbs, cholesterol, and calories. After leaving the clinic, I drove to a nearby Amish town and slid into a booth at Bird-in-Hand Family Restaurant and Smorgasbord. I asked the waitress to point out the most Amish recipe on the menu, and she suggested baked ham balls, sugar-cured and pineapple-glazed. I assumed she was referring to ham rolled into spherical shapes, as opposed to the pig's genitals. I could choose two vegetables from among a dozen or so, and both came coated in sauce. A roll and butter were placed alongside of my entrée. But even in the name of reporting, I wasn't going to subject my pancreas to the sugar assault borne by the menu's selection of homemade puddings, pies, cakes, fruit crisps, brownies, cobblers, and ice cream. The Amish disdain for frills doesn't apply to desserts, it seems. They tend to end all meals with a sugary treat, such as their trademark shoofly pie, made of molasses.

As a result, the Amish have an average BMI of 27. That's in line with the country at large, meaning it's too high. Despite this girth, they're physically fit. "The average resting heart rate among the Amish is in the sixties [that's beats per minute], even among the elderly," Sue Shaub, R.N., a clinical nurse, told me. Readings in the high forties and low fifties, rare elsewhere, are routine among the Amish, especially fieldworkers. They embody Dr. Blair's "fat but fit" hypothesis.

"Their lifestyle is what we all should be doing," says Mary Morrissey, R.N., who's been running day-to-day operations at the clinic for the past decade.

Rather than surfing the Internet and jabbing away at smart phones, the Amish are still doing the agrarian equivalent of what those ancient fishermen from British Columbia did. "My husband's a farmer, so we all work hard and we're hungry," Sally Fischer, a forty-nine-year-old Amish mother of fifteen, told me. A diet that would give an inactive person a spare tire fuels a day's work for the Amish, even if it leaves behind a few extra pounds.

I had been sitting on a wooden stool next to Sally, her gray hair showing under a bonnet, as she lay under blankets in a darkened room, hooked up to an ultrasound machine for one of Dr. Shuldiner's experiments. When the nurse stepped out, a comfortable silence settled upon two people with very different life experiences. I have no children. This woman has spawned so much life that she often calls her kids by the wrong names. I was thinking about what different lives we lead and wondering what she must be thinking about me, when she looked up from the bed. "You said your father has diabetes?" she asked. Apparently she had overheard a nurse asking me about this book.

"Yeah, he does," I said.

"My mother faced the same situation," said Sally, not a diabetic herself. "She had a sore, a black spot on the bottom of her foot, and it got bigger and bigger. The doctor said that he would have had to take her foot off. But she passed away before that had to happen. Which may have been a good thing, because at least she didn't have to suffer that."

DR. ZIMMET THINKS we need to stop thinking in terms of vulnerable populations—African Americans, Hispanics, aboriginals, or whomever—and think instead of the paucity of protected populations. Runaway diabetes is the new normal; metabolically healthy populations are fast becoming the outliers.

"There's evidence now that virtually every population in the world is vulnerable to type 2 diabetes," he says. "There is a variation in the genetic susceptibility so that, for example, Native Americans have a much higher susceptibility to diabetes than European Americans. The vulnerable groups might need only a minor degree of obesity to precipitate diabetes. If there's a lower susceptibility, it'll take more environmental influence. There's always an interplay between genes and lifestyle."

The take-home lesson: Even those with high-risk DNA, through no fault of their own, can avoid the disease. People like the aboriginal groups. People like my father and me. Sure, the headwinds can feel stiff sometimes, and pockets of turbulence are inevitable. That just means that those of us at risk must be more vigilant in avoiding the disease and more steadfast in fighting it. But with rare exceptions, no strand of DNA makes type 2 diabetes your destiny.

The Amish teach us that regular physical activity, independent of its effect on body weight, can protect against type 2 diabetes. So if you do nothing else aside from cutting back on sugar, don't sit still. You don't need to plow the fields like an Amish farmer. But whether you work behind a computer or drive a truck for a living, strive to match that level of caloric expenditure in the gym or elsewhere.

It might end up saving your life.

7

READING BETWEEN THE LINES

"[Diabetes] pills work best when used with meal planning and exercise," reads the ADA's Web site. "This way you have three therapies working together to lower your blood glucose levels." True, but two of those therapies, meal planning and exercise, can often do the job without the third. If only they were given the chance.

The emphasis at the ADA conference in New Orleans reflects the organization's priorities, with drug makers the dominant presence. Their multimedia booths resemble Hollywood sets, manned by the same sort of statuesque models who ornament auto shows. Abbott's booth is labeled "A Promise for Life." Device makers Medtronic and Johnson & Johnson are also here. Attendees can set down goodie bags and play an elaborate video game at the booth of Bristol-Myers Squibb and its partner AstraZeneca. Pastels are everywhere, a far cry from the ugly reds, purples, and blacks of diabetic decay.

Some of the medicines being hawked are lifesavers, especially for those with type 1 diabetes. Today, however, type 2s outnumber type 1s twenty to one in the United States. For the former, these drugs and devices can be thought of at least in part as damage control. But much of the damage is self-inflicted, and how much control is being achieved is an open question. What's indisputable is that type 2 diabetes continues to advance unchecked despite all the pharmacological firepower being aimed its way.

Type 2 diabetes is a chronic disease, and the complications pile up like railcars in a train wreck. That's why diabetes drug makers aren't the only ones here in the Big Easy. Abnormalities in cholesterol and blood sugar tend to go hand in hand, so Lipitor is on display. Ditto for Lyrica, an epilepsy and fibromyalgia drug that also seems to lessen diabetic nerve pain. Androgel is being repped here because 40 to 50 percent of men over the age of forty-five with diabetes have lower-than-normal testosterone levels. Colgate is here because high blood sugar can make your smile resemble that of a carved pumpkin. Orthopedic shoe and prosthetics makers, whose sales figures are helped along by diabetic amputations, have smaller booths.

THIS EMPHASIS ON drugs rather than lifestyle change, and treatment rather than prevention, is evident not only at the ADA's conference but also in its clinical practice guidelines, which have been updated annually since 2001, and periodically before that. The same sort of guidelines are issued and updated by the American Heart Association, the American Cancer Society, and the other "medical specialty groups," which accounted for 40 percent of the 2,343 sets of guidelines logged in the National Guideline Clearinghouse as of April 2008. National and international diabetes organizations publish dozens of sets of guidelines specific to diabetes, reflecting each nation's range of distinctive circumstances, including ethnicity, lifestyle preferences, and societal structure. Global diabetes guidelines aren't formally harmonized, but in talking to representatives of any number of the non-U.S. national diabetes groups, my impression is that many follow the ADA's lead.

If the ADA is "leading the fight against the deadly consequences of diabetes and fighting for those affected by diabetes," as it claims, these guidelines are their battle cry. They also tend to be closely adhered to by U.S. doctors, who nonetheless must tailor the guidelines for individual circumstances and expectations. The AAFP offers members continuing-education courses on the diagnosis and treatment of type 2 diabetes, publishes two journals (*Annals of Family Medicine* and *American Family Physician*) that periodically cover diabetes-related news, and provides members with other diabetes information. "But we also let our members know [through the member newspaper, *AAFP News Now*] about the clinical recommendations of other organizations such as the American Diabetes Association," says AAFP. "So, for example, we have directed members to the ADA's Standards of Medical Care in Diabetes."

Like most sets of guidelines, the ADA's change incrementally; most of the language carries over from year to year. They aspire to be "evidence based," evidence referring mostly to research. Committee members are expected to scour the relevant studies in the field. Thus enlightened, the committee decides how much importance each study deserves and weights them accordingly. This massive data stream is funneled and distilled into a series of written recommendations.

A government-funded task force on all clinical practice guidelines recommends dividing evidence into three "levels." Level I, randomized controlled trials, offers the most persuasive data and should be treated as such, the argument goes. Such trials would include thousands of subjects scattered across numerous clinical centers. In a diabetes-related trial, researchers might arbitrarily assign one group of prediabetics to a drug regimen and another group to a regimen of lifestyle change. A third group, called the control, might receive a placebo. Years later, the researchers could evaluate the results of the treatment groups relative to the control.

According to the government task force, less-rigorous studies should be considered but given less weight. They divide this "lesser" type of evidence into two subclasses, Level II and Level III. Level II evidence is subdivided into three subsections, from well-designed controlled trials that haven't been randomized (Level II-1) down to uncontrolled trials (Level II-3). Level III evidence can include the opinions of experts based on their clinical experience, as well as the reports of expert committees.

The ADA's evidence-based guidelines follow roughly those parameters, although their labeling scheme goes A, B, C . . . and then E. Perplexed, I half-jokingly asked them if they skip D for the same reason high-rise builders skip thirteenth floors. I was told that they go straight to E because it happens to be the first letter in *expert opinion*, although it might as well stand for *expelled*.

A group of researchers did a study that analyzed twenty-six sets of diabetes guidelines from around the world, including the ADA's. They evaluated the guidelines based on the methodologies used by the guidelines panel, rather than their content. Ideally, there should be an explicit and transparent explanation of why and how they arrived at their recommendations. Most of the guidelines fell far short, however. The researchers concluded, "The methodological shortcomings of diagnostic [guidelines] in [diabetes mellitus] raise questions regarding the validity of recommendations in these documents that may affect their implementation in practice."

Anything that doesn't fit neatly within the evidence-based hierarchy becomes, de facto, "unscientific." This is a handy way of marginalizing dissenting viewpoints. As Norman Latov, M.D., Ph.D., professor of neurology and neuroscience at the Weill Medical College of Cornell University, wrote in the *Journal of American Physicians and Surgeons*, "The writings of the founders of modern medicine, including William Harvey, Louis Pasteur, or William Osler, among others, would . . . not be considered because their contributions were not based on controlled trials." In fact, many of the most important discoveries and cures in modern medicine weren't proven through the sort of trials prized in evidence-based guidelines. Today they wouldn't make the cut.

In an e-mail exchange with me, Dr. Latov posed a hypothetical scenario: Imagine if our justice system arrived at decisions this way. Published case reports are basically dismissed in evidence-based guidelines, so eyewitness testimony would be off-limits. A similar fate would befall expert opinion, which can carry great influence in the courtroom. Fortunately the courts realize that such information indeed counts as evidence, whereas the ADA views certain trials as the only real evidence.

That raises another issue: whether such reliance on evidence-based methodologies even makes that much sense for this particular disease. "Type 2 diabetes is a nutrition-based disease, and in an area like nutrition, evidence tends to be rather soft," says Edwin Gale, M.D., professor of diabetes at Bristol University in England. "It's soft because you can't put someone on a diet and leave them ignorant of what they're eating. So while you can do a double-blind trial with tablets, you can't do it with diet."

The many-headed-dragon nature of type 2 diabetes further complicates matters. These big, lengthy trials compare only one thing to another. According to Dr. Latov, "[M]edical decision making is complex and requires consideration of many variables, including clinical presentation, severity, progression, coexisting conditions, genetic or biologic variations, susceptibility to complications, and allergies to medications. It would be impossible to design trials that compare all the options." Seldom is this more applicable than with type 2 diabetes.

"People often have to make lifestyle decisions in the absence of data from controlled trials, in which case they have to use common sense, judgment, and experience," says Dr. Latov. The dearth of well-controlled long-term studies means it takes a long time to reach conclusions, let alone change standards of care. Meanwhile the smaller studies, the ones being downplayed in the evidence-based hierarchy, are often honing in on key aspects of treatment. Unfortunately they're usually ignored.

Producing clinical practice guidelines costs money, and according to the ADA, the organization's general budget funds the development and publication of its guidelines. "We do not allow specific funding of any guideline development by any corporate entity," the ADA told me. Nonetheless drug companies subsidize much of that general budget, so they help to underwrite the formulation of guidelines that will greatly influence doctors' attitudes toward prescribing the companies' drugs. Companies whose annual support of the ADA exceeds $1 million, the highest threshold, are recognized as members of the Banting Circle Elite. For 2009, six of the seven members listed under this heading were large drug firms: Eli Lilly, Merck & Co., Novo Nordisk, Sanofi-Aventis, Solvay Pharmaceuticals, and Takeda Pharmaceuticals North America. Much of the advocacy, education, and research undertaken with those funds is important and potentially lifesaving for certain diabetic patients. But one wonders if drug-making donors are shelling out millions of dollars in hopes of adorning clinical guidelines with the sort of cold-water-splashed-in-the-face lifestyle message that could shrink demand for some of their most profitable product lines. I doubt it.

Just as drug companies are bound with the organization issuing the guidelines—the ADA in this case—separate relationships bind the guideline writers themselves with various drug makers. A 2002 *Journal of the American Medical Association* study surveyed doctors on guidelines committees and found that 87 percent had "some form of interaction" with the drug industry. This included all of the diabetes guideline writers. These relationships weren't with just one company but with more than ten, on average, for all guideline writers.

What's more, of the forty-four guidelines covered by the survey, only one set declared a personal financial interaction between a guideline writer and the pharmaceutical industry, and only one set declared no conflict of interest. So in all but two cases the guidelines offered no clue as to the existence of any relationships—despite the survey's finding that nearly 60 percent of the guideline writers had a relationship with the maker of a medical product either considered for or included in their guidelines. As the study authors noted, any influence a drug maker exerts on a guideline writer will be multiplied countless times to other doctors, the readers of those guidelines.

That influence is why this subject is so important. Yet an article in a scientific journal often undergoes more scrutiny than the published guidelines that will establish standards of care for disease affecting a large percentage of the population. "Guidelines are usually not published in the same way as original papers," says Dr. Horvath of Hungary's University of Szeged. "Quite often they are not so meticulously peer reviewed, and as we don't have guideline reporting standards similar to those for many other original papers—randomized control trials, systematic reviews, or even diagnostic accuracy studies—journal editors are generally more liberal about publishing them. There is this notion that since they are written by the 'experts,' then they are automatically correct."

In reality, guidelines should be subjected to far greater scrutiny than other papers, not rubber stamped. They are the most influential documents on clinical practice, far more important than, say, a randomized control trial. After all, guidelines have a bearing on patient management, costs, insurance reimbursements, and many other factors.

So if guideline writers and other doctors are receiving support from drug makers, what are the drug makers receiving in return? "Those relationships, which have not always been disclosed to the public, are likely to have some influence on the content of those guidelines, favoring those companies' products and services," says Eric G. Campbell, Ph.D., associate professor of medicine at Harvard Medical School.

"That's a deeply flawed system and, I think, the next big front in managing conflict of interest," says the University of Pennsylvania's Caplan, a leading medical ethicist. "It's clear that you cannot have guideline panels dominated by people who are tightly linked and beholden to industry. I'm not saying you can't have some presence, but it can't be dominant, and often it is in these panels."

On the professional practice committee for the ADA's 2010 guidelines, thirteen of the fifteen members were indeed linked to the diabetes drug industry through one or sometimes many of the following relationships: membership on speakers' bureaus, advisory boards, and other committees; research and educational funding; stock ownership; and consulting arrangements. Whether 87 percent constitutes a "dominant" presence can be debated, but the extent of industry connections at minimum is very significant. Mind you, the same connectivity holds true for the guideline committees addressing most other diseases as well.

When so many committee members have so many links to drug makers, who gets crowded out of the decision-making process? The ADA claims that its professional practice committee is "multidisciplinary." However, those fifteen members do not include a single exercise physiologist. Exercise is the single most effective tool in the prevention and treatment of diabetes, and yet it receives no direct representation. Those fifteen members may consult with exercise experts, but in the end, they call the shots. This shows you where the priorities lie.

The nearly ubiquitous interweaving of committee members and the drug industry isn't some vast conspiracy. The same specialists who end up on guideline committees also appeal to drug makers as consultants because they've risen to the top of their profession and are "plugged in." Even when a very limited potential for conflicts of interest exists, however, guidelines committees will come to reflect a certain culture. If an expert panel is convened on cholesterol, for example, the members instinctively will develop guidelines for cholesterol drugs. "The specialists who usually sit on these committees tend to move quickly into drug- or device-control of a problem rather than advocating nonmedical [that is, lifestyle] means," says Caplan.

In other words, diabetes specialists will tend to preach what they themselves practice. In their defense, the patients *they* see have often already tried and failed at lifestyle therapy. "Practicing physicians and researchers are so influential in groups such as the ADA, and those people are focused on treatment," says the Center for Science in the Public Interest's Jacobson. "There's neither a lobby nor even a natural constituency for prevention. I can see why they care more about research. It's certainly an attractive fund-raising approach."

As a check against industry relationships becoming unduly influential, you might expect the committees crafting the guidelines to be not only transparent but also subject to oversight themselves. Or, at a minimum, that an overarching protocol would steer them—guidelines for the guideline makers. Actually, no. "Historically, there has been little in the way of guiding principles for these health organizations when it comes to their guidelines," says Caplan. "And, by the way, that includes who should sit on the guideline-issuing committees."

Granted it would be virtually impossible to construct a modern-day guidelines panel free of drug company links. But it's a question of degree, especially with a lifestyle disease such as type 2 diabetes. Cancer organizations publish preventive guidelines, but after a diagnosis, treatment will require a particular medical intervention. Though working a StairMaster might help prevent cancer by keeping off excess pounds, a malignant tumor of the breast or prostate gland won't disappear after a few months of training.

Through the middle of the 2000s, little had changed regarding conflict of interest and clinical practice guidelines. A report in an October 2005 issue of *Nature* echoed the thrust of the 2002 *JAMA* study, using a slightly different methodology.

More recently there have been stirrings about addressing the conflicts of interest between doctors and drug makers. Harvard's Campbell served on an Institute of Medicine committee that produced the 2009 book *Conflict of Interest in Medical Research, Education, and Practice*, in which an entire chapter was devoted to conflicts of interest in clinical practice guidelines. The authors called for a housecleaning regarding how these committees are formed and funded. "There's now traction on this issue from a major body that lots of people pay attention to," says Niteesh K. Choudhry, M.D., Ph.D., assistant professor of medicine at Harvard Medical School and associate physician at Brigham and Women's Hospital, as well as one of the authors of the 2002 *JAMA* paper. "It seems as if we're on the cusp of something happening."

Let's hope so. New diabetes drugs are being developed all the time as demand continues to grow. The newer drugs promise more, and they usually cost a lot more, too. They also tend to have less of a track record regarding safety and real-world efficacy than the older medications they seek to replace, especially the generics. "As the price tags of these drugs grow, so does the potential for conflict of interest," says Dr. Choudhry.

LIFESTYLE CHANGE IS a better alternative than drugs for both the prevention and the treatment sides of type 2 diabetes. These behavioral modifications are universally available and free; except for those in the most dire straits, every person in the country can put down a can of soda and run around the block a few times. Which raises an interesting question: If a nondrug alternative works better than the drug therapy, shouldn't the nondrug alternative be the preferred treatment? At present, no organizing principle for guidelines committees says to take the least-invasive alternative.

So recommendations to change behavior, or lifestyle, or whatever you want to call it, tend not to appear with the frequency of medications in guidelines. When they do appear, it's usually in conjunction with a medication. Diabetes organizations seem to have lost faith in what's called step therapy, whereby a doctor would tell a patient, "Let's try this first, and then if that fails, we'll go on to something else."

In August 2006, the ADA, working in concert with the European Association for the Study of Diabetes (EASD), recommended that metformin be introduced simultaneously with lifestyle changes at the time of a diabetes diagnosis. Previously the recommendation had been to at least give diet and exercise the old college try before whipping out the prescription pad. This change was made despite the Diabetes Prevention Program, where lifestyle changes won the day in the sort of lengthy, large trial trumpeted by ADA in its evidence-based guidelines.

"Metformin is insurance for people who aren't following their diet and exercise plan," John B. Buse, M.D., Ph.D., professor at the University of North Carolina School of Medicine and a past president of medicine and science for the ADA, told another *Men's Health* writer, when asked about the decision.

The drive to insure patients against unhealthy lifestyle choices—too many calories, too little exercise—doesn't seem to work in reverse, however. Just as some patients don't follow their diet, some never fill their prescriptions for diabetes medications. Even if they do, they can easily take incorrect doses or skip them entirely, just as too much food can be eaten, a workout missed. A study conducted in Scotland and published in *Diabetic Medicine* found that one-fourth of diabetic patients who had been prescribed metformin had contraindications to its use, including kidney problems and chronic liver disease. What's more, a patient on the drug who *then* develops a contraindication has only a slim chance of going off the med.

At the time of the ADA/EASD decision, metformin was even deemed worthy of consideration for certain prediabetics. According to the edict: "In addition to lifestyle counseling, metformin may be considered in those who are at very high risk for developing diabetes (combined IFG and IGT plus other risk factors such as A1C >6%, hypertension, low HDL cholesterol, elevated triglycerides, or family history of diabetes in a first-degree relative) and who are obese and under sixty years of age." This "very high risk" scenario doesn't describe outliers but rather most prediabetics, including me, at the time of my diagnosis. Impaired fasting glucose, impaired glucose tolerance, an elevated A1C, hypertension, high triglycerides, and low HDL are the fingerprints of metabolic syndrome and therefore prediabetes. That means an awful lot of individuals who don't even have the disease yet are being handed a prescription. The only paper that should be signed at this stage is a gym membership—by the patient, not the doctor.

Yes, metformin may cost as little as $18 a month in generic form. Yes, it increases insulin sensitivity and reduces glucose production, although not as well as lifestyle change can. And, yes, metformin has fewer side effects than other diabetes drugs, but side effects should never be trivialized. The drug causes diarrhea in over half of users, nausea in up to a quarter, and less often, gas, weakness, indigestion, stomach discomfort, and headaches, perhaps in part because the drug itself has a noxious odor that some users have likened to that of a dead fish. What's more, a new study links long-term metformin use with decreased vitamin B12 absorption and hence deficiencies that worsen over time. This may result in nerve problems and elevated homocysteine concentrations, a risk factor for heart disease.

Setting aside the side effects, however, what's insidious to me is the unspoken message patients receive with their prescription: "Get used to taking diabetes drugs because that's what you're going to be doing for the rest of your life."

"When people are diagnosed [with type 2 diabetes], they're ready to make a lot of changes, but if you give them a tablet, you're saying it is not their lifestyle that is the problem," said Robert Andrews, Ph.D., consultant senior lecturer in diabetes and endocrinology at the University of Bristol in England. He was being quoted in a BBC News article. Andrews helmed a study that found one in three English diabetes patients being placed on meds prematurely. So U.S. doctors aren't alone in having an itchy trigger finger when it comes to scribbling prescriptions for diabetes drugs.

Metformin can be prescribed first and subtracted later, as the ADA suggests, but it seldom works that way. "It's more work on the part of the physician to wean somebody off metformin once they've been started on it, and there's a reluctance to do that as a result," says Dr. Stafford. "The attitude is: 'We've achieved good control of your blood sugar with the drug. Why jeopardize that?'"

You can see how this all goes down. If a type 2 diabetic starts exercising, dieting, and taking metformin as "insurance," and the exercise and diet work wonders, why mess with a successful formula, even though the drug might not be doing a damn thing? "Your treatment is a success, so let's keep doing what we're doing" is what you'll hear from doctors. They're loath to subtract metformin once lifestyle changes have kicked in because the patient must then be counted on to stay the course. So they hedge the bet.

Consider the other scenario: If blood sugar control isn't achieved, the next step is to prescribe more drugs at higher doses. So even though type 2 diabetes can be defeated without any drugs, assuming it's caught early enough, a place for drugs in the treatment regimen is assured from failure through success.

An industry that forms around a chronic disease such as type 2 diabetes can become self-perpetuating. Drug companies, hospitals, health care companies—for all of them, diabetes is not only a condition to be treated in patients, but it's also an ongoing business requiring revenue growth and margin expansion. More money can be made treating diabetes than curing it. Adopting the necessary lifestyle changes means losing a current paying customer, whereas managing symptoms by providing a drug-based therapy will keep the revenue flowing for the remainder of a diabetes patient's life, even as the quality of that life evaporates.

The question is whether the ADA is more accurately described as the spearhead in the search for a cure, as its mission states, or simply an industry trade group. The latter is closer to the truth, I would argue. What's lacking in all this is true patient advocacy. That would require seeing drugs as symbols of failure, not solutions, for type 2 diabetics.

There's a more subtle feedback loop at work, too. Doctors have tons of experience writing prescriptions for metabolic syndrome but little experience weaning patients off the same drugs. That's mostly because their treatments don't work. "Most physicians have never experienced the need to decrease medication, so they're tentative about tapering insulin, antihypertensives, and diuretics rapidly," says Mary Vernon, M.D., C.M.D., a family physician in Lawrence, Kansas, and chairwoman of the board of the American Society of Bariatric Physicians.

"All this prescribing is great for the drug and medical industries, but a short-sighted, lazy way to deal with the disease," says the Center for Science in the Public Interest's Jacobson. "Diabetes can be treated very effectively through diet and exercise. Neither the American Diabetes Association nor the American Heart Association has been a strong enough advocate for measures that help patients choose that kind of a lifestyle."

Metformin is less effective than lifestyle changes. That's been proven. But the University of Massachusetts's Braun decided to study the combined effects of exercise and metformin on insulin sensitivity. He didn't expect to find synergy of the "$1+1=3$" sort, where the combination equals more than the sum of the parts. But he figured the positive effects at least would be additive, something like $1+1=2$. Each element should bring its strength to bear, right? You could still debate the medical ethics of pushing forward an invasive option, a drug, before the noninvasive lifestyle one had been given the chance to succeed on its own. But if the effects were additive, then doctors might be justified in advising patients that the combination works better than either treatment would alone.

In the study a single bout on the exercise cycle predictably made prediabetic subjects more sensitive to insulin, the desired outcome. But when the cycling was undertaken after four weeks of treatment with metformin, exercise's beneficial effect waned. As it turns out, $1+1$ doesn't equal 2, let alone 3. Hell, it doesn't even equal 1. More like ¾. Some insurance policy that is.

I asked Braun for an explanation for how this drug might interfere with exercise's positive effects on glucose metabolism. "We're working on it," he said. "Metformin is known to increase breakdown of triglycerides to fatty acids, which we did see, and this may interfere with the uptake of glucose from the blood [caused by exercise]."

When I last spoke with him, Braun was halfway through a two-year follow-up study funded by NIH. If his initial results stand, the ADA's guideline change is undermining exercise's positive influence and disabling one of our two most potent weapons in this war.

DIET AND EXERCISE don't need pairing with prescription drugs against type 2 diabetes. They work fine without them. Nor do I need to wait for their benefits to be confirmed in any official guidelines. Those inch along, whereas I'm trying to sprint past diabetes. If I come upon a new training technique or diet tip that seems promising, I'll test-drive it in my body that week. I recently added kettlebell training to my workout regimen, and I added another 5 to 10 grams of complex carbs to my diet after extending my workouts by ten to fifteen minutes a session. I'll take my chances with this sort of experimentation, rather than waiting a decade or more for some study to be conceived, approved, funded, executed, and then evaluated by a guidelines committee funded by drug companies.

Diabetes won't wait for me; why should I wait for it? I can experiment on myself because I use lifestyle change, not drugs, to fight back. If a technique or strategy doesn't work, so what? I won't overdose on too much exercise, cauliflower, almonds, or fish oil capsules. If one thing doesn't work, I try something else until I find what does work. Then I stick with it. As Dr. Latov puts it, "We can't suspend making decisions while waiting for more studies and answers, which may never arrive."

At least not before you or a loved one is six feet under.

8

PRESCRIPTIONS FOR A DISASTER

The large supply of insulin now available has brought about its use by many physicians who are more or less unfamiliar with the clinical course of diabetes, and who are using it unnecessarily (luxury use). The use of insulin and precariously high-calorie diets to fatten a diabetic unduly, or to satisfy a gluttonous appetite, or to avoid the necessity of dieting, reveals a lack of intelligent foresight on the part of the physician as well as a lack of resourcefulness in the treatment of his patients.

W. R. Campbell and J. J. R. Macleod,
Medicine, *August 1924*

Few acts of heroism can compete with discovering a life-saving drug. Pull someone from a burning house or donate a kidney, and one life has been saved. Create an antidote to a previously incurable disease, and you can save countless lives, not only those living but also those unborn. You're not just a hero. You're practically a god.

Frederick G. Banting led the quartet of scientists who figured out how to make insulin in a lab. As the man who outsmarted type 1 diabetes, he is revered as the "founding father" of diabetes drugs. His face graced the cover of *Time* during the magazine's inaugural year, 1923, the same year he shared a Nobel Prize for his discovery. In 1934, King George V anointed him Sir Frederick. Today many events, awards, and other important diabetes-related entities bear his name. When the "greatest Canadians" were ranked on a CBC show in 2004, Banting was fourth. No less than Alexander Graham Bell (ninth) and Wayne Gretzky (tenth) ranked lower.

Banting was an unlikely rock star. A former divinity student turned surgeon, he had spent time on the battlefields of World War I removing mangled limbs from soldiers. He continued operating even after he was struck with shrapnel, earning him the British Military Cross for bravery under fire. After the war ended in 1919, he opened a medical practice in London, Ontario, and became a part-time university instructor. In late 1920, while preparing for a lecture, he read a journal article concerning the removal of dog pancreases, in an attempt to harness the source of insulin. Banting already had a keen interest in diabetes, having lost a childhood friend to the disease. The article was his eureka moment. By 2:00 A.M., he was out of bed and furiously scribbling notes that would change the course of medical history.

The tale of this medical breakthrough has been told before and never better than in Michael Bliss's *The Discovery of Insulin*, which is recommended reading. To recap, Banting, then all of twenty-nine years old, knew that the attempts made in Germany in the 1880s and elsewhere thereafter had failed because while the pancreas produces insulin, it also produces digestive enzymes. Those enzymes would destroy the insulin in the dog's pancreas, leaving the surgeon removing it with a useless blob in his hands. I'm simplifying here, but Banting's breakthrough idea was to tie up the pancreatic duct, which protected the hormone, insulin, from those digestive enzymes. He could then remove sections of the dog pancreases to pinpoint the source of insulin.

Banting shared his idea with a University of Toronto professor named J. J. R. Macleod. Despite having no research training, Banting asked if he could borrow a lab and an assistant during summer vacation. Macleod finally agreed to lend lab space—but only after multiple visits from Banting, and only for eight weeks. The assistant whose help Banting was given, a chemistry-savvy grad student named Charles Best, deserved to share in the Nobel with Banting and Macleod, according to a number of diabetes historians with whom I spoke. A biochemist and professor named James B. Collip rounded out the team; his expertise was in refining the extracts.

Over the summer of 1921, the researchers' confidence grew along with tensions inside the lab. Scientific discovery requires a strange brew of flexibility and stubbornness, and neither was in short supply. The backbiting, threats, one-upmanship, and jealousy among these outsized personalities could have provided a script for one of today's prime-time medical dramas. A higher calling underpinned all the turmoil, however. People, not dogs, were dying, and these men rushed to save them.

The breakthrough was identifying the specific endocrine cells in the pancreas, called the islets of Langerhans, that produced insulin. Banting and company produced a serum viable enough to keep a diabetic hound named Marjorie alive for seventy days. The goal, however, was producing a shot that wouldn't be toxic when injected into a human patient.

In January 1922, a fourteen-year-old boy named Leonard Thompson, gravely ill with diabetes at Toronto General Hospital, received the first shot of insulin. He had an allergic reaction, so the researchers further refined their extract and tried again. After several weeks, his blood became less acidic, and his glucose levels dropped. Young Leonard's diabetic coma relaxed its death grip. He lived to twenty-seven, when he passed away from pneumonia and diabetic complications.

As one can imagine, diabetics and their loved ones were desperate to receive a dose of this miracle cure. Yet Banting's team couldn't produce pure enough insulin in large enough quantities to satisfy the demand. Nearly two years of insulin rationing separated Leonard's first injections and large-scale production. Not until October 1923 did the drug become widely commercially available. It became a resounding success.

What drove Banting in his quest? It wasn't money. He split his Nobel check with Best, and Eli Lilly and Company, not Banting, made a fortune from insulin. Today the company trades on the New York Stock Exchange with a market value of $38 billion. Banting simply wanted to hasten worldwide access to his new wonder drug.

In 1941, at the age of forty-nine, Frederick G. Banting died in a plane crash in Newfoundland. He was on yet another mission for mankind, heading to England to help coordinate medical efforts between the Brits and North Americans during World War II.

. . .

IF ONLY THE path leading away from Banting's breakthrough had merely been a steady uphill climb to victory; instead, it's been a stumbling trek into a dark abyss, with the blind leading the blind, sometimes literally. I wonder what Sir Frederick would make of today's diabetes landscape. Maybe he would think he was looking at the carnage of a third world war.

The discovery of insulin saved many lives in the short run, but it also turned type 1 diabetes into a different sort of killer. "With the description of characteristic kidney disease in 1936, physicians increasingly realized that diabetes, far from being conquered, had been transformed insidiously from an acute to a chronic disease by insulin therapy," wrote Chris Feudtner in his book *Bittersweet*, which focuses on the history of type 1 diabetes.

Yet the main thrust of diabetes care over the last fifty years or so has been to take the pharmacological approach that spared type 1 diabetics from the 1920s onward and expand the arsenal of meds to attack a different, more widespread disease: type 2 diabetes. Medical statistics were often sketchy back then, but in 1935, roughly half a million people in the United States, or 3.7 out of every thousand, had some form of diabetes. How many had type 1 versus type 2 is impossible to say for sure. The two types hadn't even been fully differentiated medically yet, let alone the patients counted as such. But I'm guessing that most of the .5 per thousand who were under the age of twenty-five had type 1. That would put them somewhere around 13 percent of the total.

So the relative sizes of the pie slices haven't changed much; the pie has just become gigantic. Not surprisingly, type 2 diabetics, not type 1s, consume the vast majority of all diabetes drugs, a $12.5-billion-in-sales market (including insulin) in 2007. That approach hasn't solved much, working about as well as a very expensive and overmatched Band-Aid.

Nonetheless, the trend continues apace. According to a report issued at the end of May 2010 by the Pharmaceutical Research and Manufacturers of America, a record-setting 235 new diabetes medications are in the R&D pipeline. This news is championed when it should raise alarm.

Twenty-four of these drugs are for type 1 diabetes, 59 address diabetes complications, 23 are "unspecified"—and 144 target type 2 diabetes. That's right, 144 more type 2 diabetes meds, coming soon to a pharmacy near you. Or not, depending on how many patients keel over from heart attacks and such during the clinical trials. Regardless, the pipeline could be jammed with a thousand drugs, but there still won't be a high-tech fix to what is a lifestyle disease.

They've been at this for a while now. The first diabetes pills, sulfo-nylureas, came on the market in the 1950s. By acting directly on the pancreas and thus mimicking glucose, these pills prompted the pan-creas to secrete insulin. Insulin and sulfonylureas remained the chief pharmacological agents of glucose control through the middle of the 1990s, when a sea change occurred. Advances in genetic enginering would revolutionize diabetes care. In theory, that is. Onto the scene the novel compounds came, one after the other, each seemingly offering more promise than the next.

Fifteen years later, the market is filled with drugs that stimulate beta cells to secrete more insulin (sulfonylureas and meglitinides), reduce glucose in the liver (biguanides, most notably metformin; and gli-tazones), act as insulin sensitizers (à la WD-40) at the insulin receptors (see previous), interfere with the breakdown of starches and complex sugars inside the gut (alpha-glucosidase inhibitors), and mimic or otherwise affect the actions of gut hormones called incretins, which increase glucose-dependent insulin secretion (GLP-1 mimetics, DPP-4 inhibitors).

To receive FDA approval for a new diabetes drug, its maker needs to demonstrate two things: that the compound lowers blood sugar when compared to a placebo, and that it can do so safely. If a drug lowers blood sugar but also raises heart attack risk, for example, that drug theoretically won't be approved—assuming that the heart attack risk can be discerned during the approval process.

The drug's performance relative to other diabetes drugs isn't an FDA litmus test. Nor is a drug's price tag, which leads to treatments such as spending upwards of $200 per prescription for twice-daily injections of a drug made from Gila monster spit. Byetta is the brand name for exenatide, developed and commercialized by a San Diego–based bio-tech firm, Amylin Pharmaceuticals, in a collaborative alliance with Eli Lilly. Lizard spit turns out to contain a chemical compound that resem-bles a hormone found in human intestines. When released, this hormone, glucagonlike peptide-1, or GLP-1, helps glucose trigger an appropriate insulin secretion in the pancreas. The exenatide molecule resembles GLP-1 enough to fake out those receptors and thus do the same job as GLP-1. They allow it to bind—picture the fighter jet carrying Will Smith and Jeff Goldblum being allowed to dock inside the spaceship in *Independence Day*. The result: lower blood sugar.

A major selling point is that Byetta only works with glucose present, so patients run little risk of hypoglycemia while taking the drug. Ap-proved in 2005, Byetta has been a hit. Annual revenues were between $600 and $700 million from 2007 to 2009. Future growth likely hinges on an extended-release version with the same active ingredient that will need to be taken only once a week. The new drug, to be marketed as Bydureon, has been developed collaboratively with not only Lilly but also Alkermes. Unfortunately for that trio of firms, the FDA approval that was expected in mid-October 2010 wasn't forthcoming. Instead, the agency asked for an additional heart study that should push ap-proval, should it come, back to mid-2012 at the earliest. By then the market will have become even more competitive. Shares of Amylin's stock shed nearly half of their value on news of the delay. Should By-dureon eventually be approved, it will compete against its own parent drug, Byetta, as well as two GLP-1 drugs made by Novo Nordisk. Roche also has been developing a GLP-1 entry, taspoglutide, to great fanfare; it seems to outperform other drugs in many respects. But data presented at the 2010 ADA conference revealed side effects and adverse events—vomiting in reaction to the initial dose, anaphy-lactic reactions after six months—that may prevent it from coming to market.

There's another way to skin this same cat. An enzyme called dipep-tidyl peptidase-4 (DPP-4) metabolizes GLP-1, so inhibiting DPP-4 also increases plasma levels of GLP-1. Again, blood sugar drops. The first DPP-4 inhibitor drug to hit the market, Merck's Januvia, the brand name for sitagliptin, remains under patent protection until 2017, and stock analysts forecast annual sales of $4.5 billion by 2013. Novartis, Takeda, AstraZeneca, and other drug firms are taking aim on this lucrative market by developing competing products.

"Even if Januvia ends up with 75 percent of the total [DPP-IV market], that still leaves 25 percent of a $6 billion pie to be carved up," said Donny Wong, a drug industry analyst with the market research and consulting firm Decision Resources. He was being quoted at Bloomberg.com, and his verb choice was fitting, given the fate of so many diabetics who rely on pharmaceutical solutions to this disease.

THE NUMBER OF diabetes drugs available in the United States has skyrocketed over the past fifteen years. So have sales, such that 2007's total was twice 2002's. An approach to diabetes prevention and treatment whose results include a doubling in the costs of drugs every five years strikes me as being a failure on those grounds alone. But this national tragedy is only in its opening act. "Our health care system is ill-prepared to absorb the increased number of diabetics that are coming, or to provide the increased resources they'll require," says Stanford's Dr. Stafford. "Drug costs are only part of an equation that also will include end-stage ramifications, such as dialysis and kidney transplantation, that happen to diabetics fifteen or twenty years after onset of the disease."

The next generation of diabetics faces the grim prospect of those health calamities appearing in middle rather than old age. The chubby kid who turns diabetic before his senior prom? He may be getting his chest cracked open in the ER in his early thirties, not his late fifties. Both the length and intensity of care made necessary by diabetes complications will increase. Left unaltered, the current trajectory will end in a health care system crash, just as surely as blood sugar rises and falls after a couple of glazed doughnuts.

In a 2007 article on diabetes in the the *New York Times*, the author wrote, "[N]o matter what they do, most people with Type 2 diabetes get worse as the years go by. Patients make less and less insulin and their cells become less and less able to use the insulin they do produce." The expert who chimes in after that passage presents the standard recipe for failure, as if it's actually a solution: "That is why it is not un- common to start initially with diet therapy, then after a few years we need to add a drug that improves insulin sensitivity," Dr. Kahn said. [C. Ronald Kahn, M.D., is a professor of medicine at Harvard Medical School.] "Then when that drug isn't enough, we add a second drug that improves insulin sensitivity by a different mechanism. Then we add a drug that stimulates that pancreas to make more insulin."

True, working alone, a diabetes drug will often fail to achieve adequate glucose control for long. But rather than figuring out *why* the drugs aren't working, doctors reason that if one isn't enough, patients need two, or three, or a bunch. As a result, a diabetic is now prescribed only one drug less than half the time. I saw this for myself in the exhibit hall at the ADA conference, where joint ventures and combination therapies and their "+" signs abounded. Even with metformin, one-quarter of all use now involves medications that merge it with other diabetes drugs in a single product, the diabetes equivalent of an all-in-one shampoo- plus-conditioner.

While more diabetics juggle more and more drugs, the price tag of each prescription soars ever higher. In 2001, the average cost of a diabe- tes prescription was $56; in 2007, it was $76. Whereas low-cost generic versions of older diabetes medications cost $10 to $60 a month, the cost of newer drugs still under patent protection can range from $150 to $250 a month.

I asked Dr. Stafford if these expensive designer diabetes meds tend to be worth the money. "In theory, it's reasonable to suppose that while we're paying a lot more money for something like insulin glargine [sold under the name Lantus], and other forms of long-acting analogues, gly- cemic control will improve in those patients," he said. "But we don't yet have evidence that this extra money we're paying translates into better outcomes or even better control, let alone enough of either to justify the cost. We simply haven't yet proven that this is an effective use of resources." A 2009 study was more emphatic than Dr. Stafford. *Con-*

sumer Reports Health concluded that these newer, more expensive diabetes drugs are no better, no safer, and cost more than their older,
cheaper counterparts.

The same study confirmed that patients often must take more than one
diabetes drug to achieve some semblance of acceptable glucose control.

"Stacking" diabetes pills also reflects reluctance by physicians and
patients alike to begin insulin injections. CDC data show that 57 percent of diabetics treat the disease with oral medication, 14 percent with
insulin, and 13 percent with both insulin and oral medication. The remaining 16 percent of diabetics take no medications at all. Alas, some
patients have reached such an advanced stage of diabetes that insulin
may be the only tool left for achieving suitable glycemic control.

Combination therapies carry risks above and beyond the combined
list of the drugs' side effects. The actions of insulin and diabetes tablets
are highly variable. Patients end up taking large combined doses to coun-
teract their consumption of carbs, whose absorption rates within the
body also vary. The more extensive the combination of carbs and drugs,
the more potential for a mismatch between the two, and the greater
the potential for blood sugar levels bouncing up and down like a yo-yo.

The ADA's "high-carbohydrate diet necessitates industrial doses of
insulin, and . . . if they only [reduced] the amount of carbohydrate . . .
people [would be receiving] physiologic doses instead of industrial doses
[of insulin], and you wouldn't get the kind of hypoglycemia they're getting," said Richard K. Bernstein, M.D., author of *Dr. Bernstein's Diabetes
Solution*, speaking on an Internet radio show. "The whole thing is crazy,
it's shameful, and the diabetic patient is orphan."

DIABETES PRESCRIPTIONS ARE just the beginning of a diabetic's
drug regimen if the underlying problem, insulin resistance, isn't addressed. During his presentations, Health Canada's Dr. Wortman shows
a Powerpoint image listing twenty classes of drugs used to treat the
fallout of metabolic syndrome and insulin resistance. Each drug class, in
turn, contains many products. Beyond diabetes pills, drugs are prescribed

to counter hypertension (diuretics, beta-blockers, ACE inhibitors, etc.), unhealthy cholesterol levels (statins, niacin, bile-acid resins, etc.), coagulation-prone blood (aspirin), obesity (pancreatic lipase inhibitors, appetite suppressants, etc.), and erectile dysfunction. At which point, an antidepressant may be in order, too.

"Drug companies want a market in which a lot of customers need the drug or potentially could take it," says Harvard Medical School's Campbell. "Ideally, from the company's perspective, the people will take the drug continuously for a long period of time, so they're looking for a chronic condition. The company is also looking for a disease diagnosed and treated primarily by specialists. If a specialist starts a patient on a drug, the primary care doctor will tend to leave them on it. So depression, type 2 diabetes, hypertension, and cardiovascular disease are highly desirable drug markets."

The biggest problem with the drug culture surrounding type 2 diabetes is the mind-set of passive acceptance that develops among patients, like the diabetic colleague of a nutritionist I interviewed. The colleague used the insulin pump, a mechanical pancreas of sorts, small enough to attach to a belt. When they sat down for lunch, the colleague reached into her bag and pulled out a Nature Valley Crunchy Granola Bar. This woman's thought process likely went . . . *Nature Valley . . . granola . . . health food!* You might think that way; I know I used to. Marketers count on it. Twenty-five grams of carbs were listed on the wrapper, so she dialed that number into her pump, knowing she'd receive the requisite amount of insulin to handle those carbs.

The truth is that those sorts of bars are little more than granola pasted together with sugar. "I asked her why she would eat something like that if she had to inject a drug into her body to metabolize it," recalls my friend. "I said, 'Doesn't that tell you something?' She said, 'My doctor never told me that. He said to calculate my carbs and enter it into my insulin meter. All I have to do is push these buttons.'" My friend suggested to the woman that she top some cottage cheese with slivered almonds and a few berries and some Splenda for added flavor. The woman declined. After all, why not follow her doctor's orders? Why even question them, when the prescription—do as you've always done and use drugs to manage the fallout—offers such an easy way out?

Why are docs so quick to whip out a prescription pad? Direct-to-consumer marketing may bring us awkward television commercials warning against four-hour erections, but doctors are on the receiving end of the real hard sell. The "pressure to prescribe" comes from both sides in viselike fashion. Our society medicates problems as a matter of course, and people want what they've seen advertised on television and elsewhere, whether it's a new car, new phone, or new pill.

Drug makers pressure doctors to prescribe as well. That's their business, of course, to push their pills, and a used-car salesman has nothing on a highly motivated drug rep. As I wrote this passage, a headline appeared announcing that Pfizer, the world's largest research-based drug company, had been penalized $2.3 billion for its marketing of thirteen different drugs for and at unapproved uses and doses. This was the company's fourth settlement over illegal marketing practices in a decade. No diabetes drugs were singled out but several drugs with metabolic syndrome uses, including Lyrica and Lipitor, were included.

But the greatest pressure to prescribe comes from doctors' own treatment plans. The first mistake is advocating a high-carb diet. This flogs the pancreas, which tries to satisfy ever-growing demand for insulin by secreting more. That works . . . for a while, anyway. The pancreas can only keep up for so long; eventually its ability to produce insulin decreases. The shortfall leaves blood sugar at high levels, at which point the patient is prescribed a diabetes tablet, in an attempt to coax more insulin from the poor, faltering pancreas. Soon enough, one tablet can't coax out enough insulin to lower blood sugar, so the patient is prescribed a combination of tablets. Once the pancreas is burned out, insulin injections are the only recourse.

The influence of drug makers on doctors has become pervasive. Data compiled by Harvard Medical School's Campbell and colleagues and published in the *New England Journal of Medicine* showed that 94 percent of all U.S. physicians enjoy some form of relationship with the pharmaceutical industry. I asked Campbell what he meant by "relationship." "That is, they get something from these companies," he said.

"Many of the relationships revolve around the giving and receiving of industry-paid-for meals, trips to sporting events, recreational activities, having their continuing medical education paid for by companies, payments for enrolling subjects in clinical trials, large research grants, and so on." He refers to it as an underground economy of influence. "I don't think the American public has any idea that it's as deep and rich as it is," he adds. "Drug companies own medicine, medical education, and medical research in America."

The "gift exchanges" between drug makers and doctors can be creative. Campbell was sitting at an airport bar one day, waiting for a flight, when he made small talk with an attractive, extraordinarily tanned young blond woman seated next to him.

"What do you do for a living that allows you to get so much sun?" he asked.

"I play a lot of golf with doctors," she said.

"Wow, that's an interesting career," he said. "You play golf with doctors?"

"Yeah, I'm paid by a large drug company, and I travel around the country playing golf with physicians four days a week. I talk to them about the drugs, joke around with them, offer them golf tips, and then we have cocktails afterward. It's a great time!"

"What qualifications do you need to get that job?" he asked.

"I was on the golf team at Arizona State," she said.

Diabetes drugs certainly aren't immune to this phenomenon; selling them is easier than it should be, even for salespeople so driven that they often profile physicians based on personality types. A doctor could theoretically offer a counterargument to the drug reps, such as pointing out the vast superiority of lifestyle change as a therapeutic intervention. But they seldom do. "Doctors don't say diet and exercise work," says Gwen Olsen, author of *Confessions of an Rx Drug Pusher.* "Doctors look primarily to prescribe drugs."

The sales job becomes easier still when drugs are moved forward in official guidelines. "Pharma puts big money into those organizations so that they will tout their products and help promote their cures when they come out," says Olsen.

. . .

DIABETES DRUGS DON'T come with just a lot of syllables and dollar signs; they also have many side effects, too. Sulfonylureas, like insulin therapy, are known to cause weight gain. During our interview, the Oregon Health and Science University Diabetes Center's Dr. Ahmann had mentioned that even modest weight loss could greatly benefit a diabetic. That makes me wonder if the reverse scenario—*gaining* ten or fifteen pounds—wouldn't be an equally great detriment to diabetes patients.

Olsen, who sold Glucophage (a metformin brand name) for Bristol-Myers Squibb in heavily Hispanic and diabetic southwestern Texas during a fifteen-year career that ended in 2000, would ask doctors why they prescribed sulfonylureas—against which she was competing—given that it fattened up overweight diabetics. According to her, "The doctors would say, 'My patients are a hundred pounds overweight already. What difference will another ten pounds make?'"

To her, this paradox—"Hey, we're going to manage your diabetes . . . by making you even fatter!"—seemed "crazy" (her term, not mine). And like any savvy salesperson, she leveraged this inconsistency. She asked her local butcher to stuff a bag full of ten pounds of fat and brought it with her on sales rounds. Before launching into her pitch, she'd ask the doctor to hold the bag until she was done. Only after her spiel would she let the laboring doctor open the bag. "I'd say, 'This is what you're telling me is insignificant for your patients' heart and abdomen to carry around all day.'"

Weight gain is one thing, but if there's one side effect that shouldn't come from a diabetes drug, it's an increased risk for cardiovascular disease and heart attacks. After all, the majority of diabetics die this way, so any drug that raises those odds would seem to be problematic, to say the least.

In August 2007, I was in Chicago, attending the Bears' summer camp to write a profile of one of their star players for *Men's Health*. Driving back to my hotel after practice, I listened to a doctor on the radio being grilled about a study published in May of that year in the

New England Journal of Medicine. The interview concerned the Glaxo-SmithKline drug Avandia, the brand name for rosiglitazone, which lowers blood sugar by making tissues more sensitive to insulin. The FDA had approved Avandia in 1999 as a type 2 diabetes treatment, solo or in combination with other oral meds. Business boomed. By 2006, annual sales had reached $3 billion. Avandia had become the top-selling oral med for diabetes in the world.

However, when the results of forty-two different trials were pooled in a new "study of studies"—the one being discussed on the radio—those taking the drug were found to have a 43 percent higher risk of heart attack and a 64 percent higher risk of a cardiovascular-related death than study participants not taking the drug.

Rosiglitazone tends to be prescribed to patients already considered to be at high risk for heart attacks. What's more, since the trials being pooled lasted only twenty-four to fifty-two weeks, the results suggested that the drug might be capable of provoking a heart-related death after relatively brief exposure.

Why rosiglitazone had this effect remains an unanswered question. The drug's label says that some patients who take it may experience an increase in LDL cholesterol levels. That certainly wouldn't be heart-helpful. "Several other properties of the drug may contribute to adverse cardiovascular outcomes," the study reads. "Rosiglitazone and other thiazolidinediones are known to precipitate congestive heart failure in susceptible patients." It went on to note that the drug might raise the risk of a condition, called myocardial ischemia, in which the heart receives insufficient blood flow.

According to the study authors, the data begged for a comprehensive evaluation to clarify the cardiovascular risks. They urged doctors to weigh the risks of rosiglitazone before prescribing it to type 2 diabetics.

On November 14, 2007, six months after the meta-analysis was published, the FDA announced that GlaxoSmithKline had agreed to update its boxed warning with new language cautioning against the potential increased risk of heart attack. No doubt in part as a result, the drug's sales were down 27 percent in 2007. At the agency's behest, a study was initiated to compare Avandia's safety with its main competitor, Actos (pioglitazone), made by Takeda. Since then, an internal debate has raged within the FDA as to whether that trial should even continue, considering Avandia's known heart risks. The results of a lengthy Senate investigation into Avandia, released in February 2010, scolded Glaxo-SmithKline for not warning consumers sooner about Avandia's heart risks.

In May 2010, GlaxoSmithKline reached its first legal settlements, $60 million worth, with seven hundred plaintiffs who contended that the drug can cause heart attacks and strokes. Analysts estimate the company will pay out more than $1 billion in Avandia-related claims.

An exposé in the *New York Times* on July 12, 2010, reported that GlaxoSmithKline and its predecessor, SmithKline Beecham, had cherry-picked data concerning Avandia, rather than reporting the damaging results of its own studies, going back as far as 1999. Apparently the goal had been to obscure those heart risks, which would later emerge in the meta-analysis done by an outsider. "With Avandia, GlaxoSmithKline has done more than hide trial data," wrote the author. "An F.D.A. reviewer who closely examined a landmark Avandia clinical trial called 'Record,' found at least a dozen instances in which patients taking Avandia suffered serious heart problems that were not counted in the trial's tally of adverse events, mistakes that further obscured Avandia's heart risks."

Later that same week, a thirty-three-member advisory panel to the FDA weighed in on the drug's fate. A plurality of twelve members voted to pull Avandia from the market. Seven members said it should remain in pharmacies but with stronger warnings about the heart risks. Ten members echoed the call for stronger warnings but supported tight sales restrictions as well. Three members voted for the status quo. A final member abstained. Sorting it all out and making a final decision would be FDA Commissioner Margaret A. Hamburg, although, if you take Avandia, the decision ultimately rests with you. After all, it's your heart.

The ADA responded predictably to the panel's vote. It took a let's-wait-and-see approach. It gave the drug and its maker, one of its Banting Circle benefactors, the benefit of the doubt. And its statement was made jointly with another organization. "The worst outcome would be to not treat diabetes properly, thereby risking its complications," said Daniel Einhorn, M.D., president of the American Association of Clinical Endocrinologists, in a joint ADA/Endocrine Society statement.

In September 2010, regulators in the United States and Europe issued a joint announcement that will drastically reduce Avandia use. In Europe, the door was slammed shut on new Avandia prescriptions. In the United States, the door was left slightly ajar. Only those diabetes patients who have failed a range of other treatments, and who have been alerted to the heart risks of Avandia, can receive a prescription.

THE UPROAR OVER Avandia wasn't the only troubling link between diabetes drugs and heart failure in 2008. In February, when I was about to complete the *Men's Health* feature that inspired this book, the National Heart, Lung, and Blood Institute discontinued part of a large study using drug-heavy glucose-lowering strategies. A scan of preliminary data showed that intensively lowering blood glucose to near-normal levels produced a 22 percent increase in deaths versus a less-intensive approach. As a safety precaution, the intensive-treatment study arm was discontinued eighteen months before the study's original 2009 ending date.

The trial was called Action to Control Cardiovascular Risk in Diabetes (ACCORD). The "action" basically meant taking lots of drugs. Beginning in 2001, 10,251 type 2 diabetics between the ages of forty and seventy-nine enrolled in the trial. On average, they had spent a decade as diagnosed diabetics. Among other requirements, study participants either had to have experienced a cardiac event in the past or be at high risk for cardiovascular disease. ACCORD was designed to compare varying degrees of drug intervention; it didn't pit drugs versus lifestyle change.

The intensive-study arm was included because past studies suggested that lowering blood sugar to nearly normal might make type 2 diabetics less prone to cardiac events. The goal established for them was an A1C below 6 percent, the sort of level found in nondiabetics.

The less-aggressive standard treatment aimed for a figure of 7 to 7.9 percent, still suggestive of diabetes, although not terrible. The A1C of the average U.S. type 2 diabetic is 8.2 percent.

A1C scores below 6 percent were to be achieved through high doses of multiple oral medications and insulin. Slightly more than half the participants in the intensive-approach group were taking three oral meds along with their insulin. In contrast, only 16 percent of those in the standard-treatment group took such an extensive array of diabetes drugs.

In only four months, the average A1C in this group fell from 8.3 percent to 6.7 percent. By that yardstick, the aggressive approach worked. But the higher death rate in the intensive group suggested that, at a minimum, a treatment regimen this aggressive may not be appropriate for those older, long-standing type 2 diabetics already showing signs of heart disease.

The biggest surprise may be that this came as such a big surprise. "There's always been this question of whether the elderly should lower their blood sugar when their coronary disease is fairly well along," says Dr. Barnett. "It's not very good to throw them into low blood sugars, and does it do much good, anyway?"

Why might using drugs to almost coerce the metabolic systems of patients with cardiovascular disease into tight blood sugar control actually harm them, perhaps even kill them in certain instances? "There's been a concern raised that low blood sugars in patients with cardiovascular complications could increase the risk of cardiovascular events because when you have a low blood sugar, your body releases hormones that increase stimulation to the heart," says Mary-Elizabeth Patti, M.D., an investigator and adult endocrinologist at Joslin Diabetes Center in Boston.

In addition to suffering more deaths than expected, members of the intensive-strategy group experienced side effects such as hypoglycemic episodes, fluid retention, and weight gain. In fact, 30 percent of the ACCORD participants gained twenty-two or more pounds during the study. Again, this side effect seems like a really, really bad trade-off for a type 2 diabetic.

Treating any single study, including ACCORD, as the last word on aggressive blood sugar lowering would be a mistake. But this was the sort of ambitious, long-term study whose result will wield great influence in the diabetes community for years to come. The findings can't be easily dismissed.

In the aftermath, many hypotheses were ventured. A popular one among diabetologists suggested that the blame lay with severe hypoglycemic episodes. Yet while hypoglycemia was indeed associated with a higher risk of death in both study arms, subsequent analyses failed to pinpoint this factor as explaining the difference in death rates between the two cohorts. The volatility that might result from such pharmacological firepower involves more than just selected hypoglycemic episodes of great severity, however. That's merely one pole. Those running the studies were looking at averages, but how often were the subjects actually at that number? No systematic continuous glucose monitoring was conducted in ACCORD, so the researchers can't know the extent of the variability and volatility. A1C scores do not capture that data.

A U.K. study published in the *Lancet* calls further into question the notion of using aggressive, insulin-led drug treatments to lower A1C scores in diabetics. Of the nearly 50,000 diabetic patients being studied, those with the highest *and* lowest A1Cs had higher death rates than those whose score fell in between. What's more, death rates were nearly 50 percent higher among those whose regimen included taking insulin, compared to those taking oral meds but not insulin.

"It all goes to show they're missing the forest for the trees by treating the symptoms rather than addressing the basic cause of high blood sugar," says the University of Connecticut's Volek, who points to carb-induced insulin resistance as that cause. "I've never thought that pumping people full of insulin, even in an attempt to control blood glucose, would be a good thing."

DIABETES DRUGS AREN'T the only meds exerting a negative long-term effect on glucose metabolism while producing unwanted side effects. "People with diabetes are usually on blood pressure medicines, arthritis medicines, cholesterol medicines, and they all have little annoying side effects that start to add up," the ADA's Dr. Buse has been quoted as saying.

Annoying is one word for it when a drug prescribed for hypertension is actually setting the stage for diabetes. For more than a decade prior to my prediabetes diagnosis, I had been popping one of those pills mentioned by Dr. Buse. Hydrochlorothiazide is part of a drug family called the thiazide diuretics, our nation's first line of drug defense against hypertension. Here, as well as in Europe, guidelines recommend that if patients with uncomplicated hypertension need a drug, they take these pills first. Doctors had prescribed it for me as my blood pressure became hypertensive during my early thirties.

Diuretics are water pills; they make you pee. The resulting loss of fluid and sodium should lower blood pressure. The most effective of the three types of diuretics used to lower blood pressure are thiazides, which may also widen blood vessels, another blood-pressure-lowering effect. Their effects are also longer lasting than those of other diuretics.

Doctors prescribe thiazide diuretics as if they're handing out candy on Halloween night. There are about ten different versions currently on the market, and total sales of thiazides and related agents registered more than $42.5 million in 2005.

Side effects of thiazides worth considering include fluid loss and even occasional dehydration. That's worrisome because staying properly hydrated is essential for overall health. Sodium isn't the only electrolyte flushed out by diuretics; potassium and magnesium go as well. Magnesium levels are notoriously low among diabetics.

"What's not widely known but nonetheless well established are the lipid consequences of diuretics," says William R. Davis, M.D., a cardiologist in Milwaukee, Wisconsin, and the author of *Track Your Plaque*. "There's a drop in HDL [healthy cholesterol], a rise in triglycerides, and a rise in the number one cause for heart disease: small-size LDL [unhealthy cholesterol] particles. It varies by individual, but the effect can be substantial."

The thiazides have an even more intimate connection to diabetes, and it's an insidious one. It was only after my appointment with Dr. H. that I learned that these medications have been shown to worsen glucose metabolism. By taking this medication, had I been helping type 2 diabetes set up shop inside my body without even knowing it?

As I read about this phenomenon, I found myself scratching my head. For starters, the negative effect of thiazides on glucose metabolism was first noted in 1959 and has been confirmed repeatedly, including a review of fifty-nine relevant drug trials that established a "strong relationship" between diuretics and a rise in blood glucose. The thiazides make the beta cells in the pancreas less sensitive to glucose, so the pancreas doesn't secrete sufficient insulin to direct enough blood glucose into cells.

This process doesn't unfold overnight. Studies find no change in glucose metabolism after a year but significant deterioration after about six. No one with whom I spoke disputed the underlying cause and effect—just the degree of the effect, and the trade-offs.

"If you look at populations whose blood pressure is being treated with other drugs versus treated with thiazides, the latter have an increased chance of having diabetes," says Dr. Ahmann, adding that the problem was more pronounced back when thiazides were dispensed in higher doses than they are now. The difference today, he said, is that doctors don't prescribe a dosage greater than 12.5 to 25 milligrams for diabetics. Before, patients took 50 to 100 milligrams.

Dr. Ahmann contends that taken in today's lower amounts, thiazides don't disturb glucose metabolism. "Small doses are important in trying to control blood pressure, and blood pressure has a big impact on complications in people with diabetes," says Dr. Ahmann. "So we endorse small doses of the thiazides. Just not the big doses."

The ADA's Dr. Deeb agrees that when thiazides are dosed correctly, the potential benefit outweighs the risk. I had asked him: If I were taking a thiazide and my blood sugar was high, should I stop taking the drug? "No, what you need to do is control your blood pressure, too, and there may be other, more powerful reasons to take it," he said. "There are some pretty powerful studies, particularly in African Americans, that some drugs work better for blood pressure, so you need to be careful that all three variables are controlled: blood sugar, blood pressure, and cholesterol."

What if insulin resistance lies at the root of high blood sugar, blood pressure, and cholesterol, with hypertension a signal that ever-increasing insulin blasts and blood sugar swings are stressing the cardiovascular system? High blood pressure may be an early warning of insulin resistance, one that often appears well before high blood sugar. But in attempting to treat the early warning sign, doctors and drug makers help worsen your blood sugar until it turns diabetic. All these drugs suppress symptoms; they don't fix anything or change the metabolic outcome. If pots are boiling over on the stove, why not turn off the burners rather than trying to keep lids on the situation as they rattle loose?

Given my family history and medical state, taking any drug that hindered my glucose metabolism even a bit seemed like a terrible idea. Why give type 2 diabetes any sort of helping hand? At my next appointment, I raised the thiazide issue with my doctor. If you're in the same boat I was in, consider doing the same. I suggested to my doc that I be switched to an ACE inhibitor, the one whose effects on blood sugar are relatively benign. He agreed.

I'd later find out that Australia has changed its guidelines to make ACE inhibitors their first pharmacological line of defense against hypertension. The reason: because thiazide diuretics raise the odds of type 2 diabetes. The United States and Europe haven't followed suit.

Eventually I would end up tossing my bottle of ACE inhibitors, too, as my blood pressure normalized by itself when I cut way back on my carbs. Dr. Davis says he sees this effect all the time in his practice.

UNFORTUNATELY, THE UNITED STATES finds itself with a huge number of type 2 diabetics whose disease is long-standing. For them, the drugs are now a necessary evil. "As a clinician, your best result is achieving good glycemic control without insulin," says Stanford's Dr. Reaven. "But not using insulin if you can't achieve that would be a mistake. High glucose concentrations are a potent factor for kidney disease, eye disease, and damage to other small blood vessels. So if the hyperglycemia requires insulin, you really must use it. Otherwise, you're substituting a hypothetical problem [the effects of excessive insulin production] for a real one [the effects of high blood sugar]."

If only more patients knew how to alter their lifestyle to lower high blood sugar without insulin or other diabetes drugs, or how to avoid high blood sugars in the first place. "That we do devote so many resources to diabetes medications is a function of how we prioritize different activities within the health care system," says Dr. Stafford. "We value the medications and their ability to prevent complications, and the medications certainly do that. But at the same time, we're devaluing the roles of prevention and earlier intervention by physicians."

And when doctors do intervene, the course of action is too often misguided.

"Very few in the medical profession are guiding patients in the right direction," says Dr. Bernstein. This echoes the feeling I had upon leaving Dr. H.'s office as a freshly minted prediabetic, namely that I was alone in trying to fend off the disease. That shouldn't be a prerequisite to staying healthy, especially since most people don't have dozens of health experts at their disposal, the way a journalist does. How do those people even stand a fighting chance against this deadly disease?

It may sound as if doctors and drug makers are in cahoots to destroy your health, but that isn't the take-home message. Drugs can play a critical role in the treatment of type 2 diabetes—once significant lifestyle change has been fully, not halfheartedly, explored. Prevention, early detection, and then an immediate counterassault through lifestyle modification are the antidotes to type 2 diabetes. The earlier the intervention occurs, the better the outcome in most cases.

9

PUTTING THE "DIE" IN DIET

f Dr. Joslin had it right in the early 1900s, why have we been heading in the opposite direction ever since? How have we turned type 2 diabetes from being a medical oddity into an epidemic?

As complicated as any public-health problem inevitably is, the diabetes epidemic boils down to two main variables. The first variable is the decline in physical activity over the past century, to the extent that one in four Americans engage in nothing that could reasonably be deemed physical activity. They are couch potatoes, firmly rooted. Sixty percent of Americans don't engage in enough activity to derive any health benefit.

The second factor is the increase in the consumption of calories, particularly carbs. Many are in the dark about what they feed their own body. When researchers ask people to venture a guess, and then monitor their diet, the subjects are usually eating more than three times the number of carb grams that they thought they were. No wonder per capita sugar consumption in the United States has risen from 5 pounds in the latter part of the nineteenth century to 25 pounds in the latter part of the twentieth century to 160 pounds today.

Nor do people realize that they've been steered in this direction. For the groundwork to be laid for the dietary portion of the equation, seemingly unrelated forces needed to coalesce:

- The U.S. government's dietary recommendations, which promoted carbohydrates as the foundation of a healthy diet, aka the food pyramid, throughout the twentieth century
- The U.S. government's farm policy, which over the same span promoted the provision of inexpensive calories, namely, carbohydrates
- A misguided belief, fostered around the mid-twentieth century, that saturated fat is the main culprit in heart disease
- A misguided emphasis on one consequence of type 2 diabetes (heart disease) rather than its underlying cause (insulin resistance)

Here's how it all started.

To figure out the carbohydrate content of a food that might be given to a patient in one of his metabolic wards, Dr. Joslin referenced the work of a Yale-educated USDA food chemist named Wilbur Olin Atwater. Using an instrument of his own invention—the calorimeter— Atwater quantified the carbohydrates, protein, and fat content of foods, thereby undertaking the first scientific study of food composition. His food lists were published in 1906 under the catchy title "The Chemical Composition of American Food Materials, Bulletin No. 28, Revised Edition." By coupling these lists with more diabetes-specific data from the Connecticut Agricultural Experiment Station, Dr. Joslin was able to fine-tune the diets he prescribed for his patients.

Atwater's work was the prototype of what later became known as the food guides, and then later, the *Dietary Guidelines for Americans*. Coincidentally Atwater's personal dietary views favored protein, beans, and vegetables, healthy choices then, and now. He also thought Americans needed to exercise more.

The championing of protein and fat by Dr. Joslin and a few like-minded medical professionals may have served diabetics well, but the rest of America was consuming meals high in carbs. They did so for the same reason many people consume them today—because meat and fish were too expensive. At the turn of the century, most working-class Americans spent half their income on food, far more than the 13.3 percent spent on average today. A high-carb diet was all they could afford back then.

It was no accident that carbs were so inexpensive. In attempting to support farmers who were being hit harder than most by the ensuing downturn, government policy had set in motion a process that would shift consumption patterns toward carbs. The initial farm bill, the Agricultural Adjustment Act, was passed in 1933, with an eye toward using subsidies and other support mechanisms to support certain crops to the exclusion of others. Wheat, corn, rice, and four other products were anointed as commodity crops, and through various means, the U.S. government began to support their pricing. Everything else, including fruits and vegetables, was deemed a specialty crop and received no such assistance.

Supporting prices paid to farmers for corn, especially, had the short-term effect of raising food prices. But in the long term, this reorientation centered U.S. agricultural production on providing cheap calories. "Government farm programs once designed to limit production and support prices (and therefore farmers) were quietly rejiggered to increase production and drive down prices," wrote author Michael Pollan in *The Omnivore's Dilemma*. Adjusted for inflation, the prices paid to farmers for their crops declined at a 1 percent annual rate during the twentieth century, to the benefit of consumers. Whereas in 1950 Americans spent 22 percent of their disposable income on food to be prepared at home, that figure had fallen to 7 percent by 2000. Food was growing cheaper and people were eating out more. The net result was Americans fattening up like so much livestock.

Dietary recommendations are a zero-sum game, no matter who formulates them; as the percentage of one macronutrient rises, another's must fall. If carbs were going to become the cornerstone of the American diet and an engine of economic growth in the heartland, something else would have to become the villain.

Enter fat.

After the discovery of insulin, diabetic diets zigzagged. High-carb

diets, low-carb diets, "free" diets, and other approaches fell in and out
of fashion with the frequency of hemlines during the first half of the
twentieth century. But in 1950, when the ADA issued its first formal
dietary recommendations, diabetics were steered toward fare different
from the meals filling the plates of the rest of the United States. The
ADA's first diabetic diet, formulated in concert with the American Dietetic Association and the U.S. Public Health Service, consisted of 40
percent carbs, 20 percent protein, and 40 percent fat. This carb allocation fell below what nondiabetic America was consuming, and it made
sense to differentiate diabetic diets from the normal American diet,
which wasn't particularly healthy. Food rationing was still a fresh mem-
ory, so the pendulum swung hard the other way. Dinner was cooked
and eaten at home more often than not, and meals based around comfort foods such as tuna casserole, meat loaf "frosted" with mashed potatoes, lasagna, Swedish meatballs, mashed potato "volcanoes," "pigs in
blankets," and desserts tended to be high in carbs, protein, fat, cholesterol, and calories.

But the future of the American diet—and the real trouble brewing
for America's glucose metabolism—can be seen with benefit of hindsight, given food chains that came into being during the 1950s. Dunkin'
Donuts appeared in 1950, Taco Bell and Jack in the Box in 1951, Den-
ny's in 1953, Burger King in 1954, and McDonald's and Kentucky Fried
Chicken in 1955. Gaining weight was suddenly convenient. Studies
tracking the eating habits of young adults not only find that frequent
fast-food diners gain more weight than less-frequent diners over the
long haul, but that frequent diners are also much more prone to having
insulin resistance and the rest of the metabolic syndrome.

Another kind of convenience—the need to produce a scapegoat for
heart disease—would also help set the stage for a diabetes epidemic.
The U.S. medical establishment, worried about rates of heart disease,
began championing a cause-and-effect relationship with dietary fat and
cholesterol on the one hand and cardiovascular disease on the other.
Leading experts decided that since diabetics most often die from heart
disease, prevention and treatment should focus on heart health rather

than on diabetes itself. The dietary advice for protecting the heart was to eat less fat and more carbs. The emphasis on heart health rather than glucose metabolism as the key to managing the disease persists. In a major piece on diabetes published in the *New York Times*, the author, talking about a forty-three-year-old diabetic man who had suffered a heart attack, wrote: "[I]n focusing entirely on blood sugar, Mr. Smith ended up neglecting the most important treatment for saving lives—lowering the cholesterol level. That protects against heart disease, which eventually kills nearly everyone with diabetes."

Everyone, including diabetics, should watch their LDL. But to say that lowering LDL is *the* single key to saving the lives of diabetics is absurd. The key is mending the underlying cause of diabetes: insulin resistance, which leads to elevated blood sugar. I can't think of another major disease where the approach to treatment focuses on something besides that disease.

What's more, the connections among fat, cholesterol, and heart disease that have underpinned this focus aren't well founded. (Gary Taubes's book *Good Calories, Bad Calories* offers a wonderful rendering of this disconnect.) Blood-borne cholesterol and heart disease share an association, but not necessarily one of cause and effect. Half of all heart attacks strike people with normal cholesterol; half of those whose cholesterol is elevated show no signs of heart disease. There are at least five different versions of the unhealthy cholesterol, LDL; the healthy kind, HDL, has at least three. Every subgroup affects heart health in a different way.

Trying to link blood-borne cholesterol with the cholesterol in, say, last night's steak dinner further muddies the water. You could eat a cholesterol-packed diet and still have normal or even low cholesterol; I could excise every ounce of known cholesterol from my diet and still have heart-attack-waiting-to-happen readings. The human body seeks homeostasis; it tends to ramp up production of what it doesn't receive, and manufacture less of what it does. On balance, blood cholesterol scores seem to reflect the stuff produced in the liver more than they reflect dietary cholesterol.

But Americans were suffering high rates of heart disease, so Congress sprang into action by launching nine years of hearings. The Select Committee on Nutrition and Human Needs was formed in 1968 and overseen by Senator George McGovern. Most politicians don't know much about nutritional science, so they summoned a flock of scientists and medical experts, many of whom fingered dietary fat as the main cause of heart disease. Evidence to the contrary was invisible during the deliberations.

Back then the idea that fat could cause heart disease resonated with people, the South Dakota politician included. It resonates with people today. You trim some fat from a piece of meat, picture it clogging your arteries, and think, *Aha! Heart attack waiting to happen. Fat's the problem*. Anyone can understand that.

Only it doesn't work that way.

With the issuance of the McGovern committee's *Dietary Goals for the United States* report in 1977, the procarb crowd had a congressional mandate in hand. As 1970s cultural signposts went, dietary fat became as unpopular as disco. Food producers, however, rejoiced, realizing they could turn this nationwide fear of fat into new product lines.

The "healthier" alternative spawned a low-fat fever that swept over America's supermarkets, airwaves, and bookstores. There was the 1984 *Time* magazine cover showing two eggs, sunny side up, and a slice of bacon arranged into a frown below the word *cholesterol* in block letters. There was Australian housewife Susan Powter imploring Americans to "stop the insanity" and eat anything you want—as long as you avoid fat. Sugary cereals for the kids? No fat, no problem! Alerted to this dietary danger everywhere they turned, moms and dads hell-bent on keeping their families and themselves safe from a heart attack were scooping up low-fat versions of everything. Unfortunately, many of these products replaced that fat with the real villain, sugar.

Health organizations mimicked the feds. As the century progressed, the ADA steered away from its 1950 stance and advised diabetics to eat *more* carbs. In 1986, they recommended a seismic shift, elevating carbs to 60 percent or less of total calories while lowering fat to 30 percent or less. Protein could range from 10 to 20 percent.

The McGovern report also paved the way for the *Dietary Guidelines for Americans*, to be issued every five years, beginning in 1980. In 1992, these bullet points became the bricks for building the Food Guide Pyramid, which beamed the low-fat message into psyches of all ages. Fat stood at the pyramid's pinnacle, along with oils and sweets, meaning that they were to be consumed in the smallest amounts.

Obesity and type 2 diabetes rates continued to skyrocket. Alarmed, nutritionists at the Harvard School of Public Health realized that the government's carb-based food pyramid was making the situation worse; it was, in fact, upside down. Wrote one of the Harvard experts, Walter C. Willett, M.D., in his 2001 book *Eat, Drink, and Be Healthy*, "At best, the USDA's Pyramid offers wishy-washy, scientifically unfounded advice on an absolutely vital topic—what to eat. At worst, the misinformation contributes to overweight, poor health, and unnecessary early deaths." The Harvard team designed their own version of the pyramid, inverting the positions of refined carbs and fats. Their concept was introduced in Willett's book.

With more than two-thirds of the country overweight five years into the new millennium, the USDA realized that, indeed, the pyramid needed to do some remodeling. "With its layering of food groups, the original pyramid may not have been the best conveyor of dietary guidance, and that's why it was overhauled," Robert C. Post, Ph.D., deputy director of USDA's Center for Nutrition Policy and Promotion, told me during a phone interview.

Dr. Bernstein put it more bluntly: "The Food Guide Pyramid pointed the American people in exactly the wrong direction. It made people fat and caused type 2 diabetes."

Post says that dietary guidance reflects "the best science at the time," implying that it's easy to use today's research to pick apart yesterday's guidance mistakes. Which is true. Indeed, MyPyramid, which debuted in 2005, corrected the egregious mistake of making the foundation a bunch of foods that become sugar when digested. This new "translation tool," in USDA parlance, arrays five food groups along the bottom: grains, vegetables, fruits, milk, and meat and beans. For good measure, a figure is shown jogging up the pyramid's stairs.

The pyramid itself no longer contains much information; it's more of a signpost. Learning more requires logging on to the USDA's Web site, which allows visitors to apply Uncle Sam's dietary advice to their own diets, depending on factors such as age and activity level. "The pyramid is kind of irrelevant, especially since they stripped it of any information," says the Center for Science in the Public Interest's Jacobson.

In an age when dietary advice proliferates across the Internet and elsewhere, does anyone even pay attention to MyPyramid and its recommendations? Apparently. In late May 2010, this Web tool attracted 9.6 million visitors and 36.3 million page views a year to date. Clearly Americans give credence to what their government says about what to eat.

Post is a thoughtful, articulate advocate for the USDA's efforts to improve dietary guidance. But even he conveys no sense of diabetes being the predictable outgrowth of how our nation eats. "I'm not necessarily aware of a link between the availability of carbohydrate-based foods and the potential for diabetes," he told me. "And the grain food group includes more than sugars. It includes whole grains and complex carbohydrates, which contribute dietary fiber."

Even though the Harvard School of Public Health noted some improvements in the USDA's 2005 updating of the guidelines, it again hammered USDA on this crucial point. "The [2005] guidelines suggest that it is fine to consume half of our grains as refined starch," its nutritionists wrote. "That's a shame, since refined starches, such as white bread and white rice, behave like sugar. They add empty calories, have adverse metabolic effects, and increase the risks of diabetes and heart disease."

As Post points out, the dietary guidelines are aimed at helping the general population balance their daily diets. They're not designed to manage type 2 diabetes. But maybe they should be crafted, at least in part, to prevent insulin resistance. After all, the CDC now predicts that should current trends continue, as many as one in three U.S. adults will have full-on diabetes by 2050.

"For the general U.S. population, the carbohydrate level should be much lower than what's currently recommended," says Raab. Beyond that, emphasis should also be placed on shifting carb consumption toward those that enter the bloodstream slowly rather than quickly. A USDA spokesman told me that incorporating the glycemic index into the guidelines was seriously considered but ultimately rejected during the advisory committee's deliberations for 2005.

In their June 15, 2010, "Report of the Dietary Guidelines Advisory Committee," which will inform the 2010 *Dietary Guidelines for Americans*, the thirteen-member committee concluded, "When selecting carbohydrate foods, there is no need for concern with their glycemic index or glycemic load." But if you're among the one in three U.S. adults with diabetes or prediabetes, then you are exceedingly concerned with the glycemic index and load of your carb foods. High GI carbs will spike your blood sugar in a heartbeat, and that's not healthy for anyone.

For dietary guidance specific to their disease, diabetics should turn to an agency within the U.S. Department of Health and Human Services, or to the American Diabetes and American Dietetic associations, Post advises. However most of these organizations have decided that what's good for everyone else is also good for diabetics. Whole grain bread? Diabetics should rely on such foods, we're told. The fact that this bread doesn't dissolve into glucose quite as fast as white bread doesn't make it healthy for diabetics. USDA defers to the two ADAs—which largely base their dietary guidelines on the USDA's. What's lacking in this feedback loop is any sense of accountability. Unfortunately, the dietary paradigm that's churning out legions of diabetics isn't the cure for the situation it helped create.

The problem is that as fat intake shrank gram by gram in the American diet, American waistlines grew inch by inch. The obesity rate climbed from 15 to 31 percent between 1971 and 2000. This was inevitable: carbs promote hunger, whereas protein and fat satisfy it. And all too often, the words *reduced fat* on a label were interpreted as low calorie, when they were code for *slightly* less terrible for you. Even today, switching from the original Cracker Jacks to the reduced-fat version drops the calories from 120 to 110, with the same 28 grams of blood sugar–skyrocketing carbs included in the mix. So you can eat five boxes with impunity from weight gain, right? That's only one of the nearly countless foods whose reduced-fat versions produce only negligible calorie reductions per serving. A serving of regular Oreo cookies has 160 calories and 7 grams of fat. The reduced-fat version has 150 calories and 4.5 grams of fat. Each one contains 14 grams of sugar. Switching from one version to the other accomplishes little of nutritional value, and it may encourage you to eat even more.

Here's the truth: Unless accompanied by a heavy carb load, fat shouldn't make you fat. Carbs are the perpetrator of our obesity and diabetes epidemics. Half a century of fat restriction wasn't merely a major distraction from what should have been the focus: carbs. Dollar for dollar, this low-fat fixation may well have been the most expensive public-health blunder in U.S. history.

If this fat phobia was misguided for healthy Americans, imagine how it played out for the glucose intolerant. No wonder we're now facing an epidemic.

USDA GUIDELINES DON'T form in a vacuum. The department's constituencies include not only American consumers but also food producers. U.S. farmers grow a lot of grain, and commerce being commerce, much of it must enter the food supply. What's more, many carb-centric food makers possess deep pockets. Like any industry leaders, they make their voices heard in the nation's capital.

In fact, every interested party is given the chance to speak its mind. The USDA solicits public comments in the months leading up to the aforementioned advisory committee report, the one that foretells the content of the actual guidelines. I read through nearly a thousand comments provided for the 2000 and 2005 guidelines, and some were simply the opinions of average citizens like you and me.

Most comments, however, came from the food industry and health organizations, reflecting the meteoric impact of these guidelines on everything from commerce to medicine. Carbs are well spoken for. For the 2005 guidelines, often-lengthy, in-depth comments were received from:

- General Mills
- The USA Rice Federation
- The Sugar Association
- The American Beverage Association
- The North American Millers' Association
- The Snack Food Association
- The Foundation for the Advancement of Grain Based Foods
- The W. K. Kellogg Institute
- The National Milk Producers Federation
- The Wheat Foods Council
- The National Restaurant Association
- The National Pasta Association
- The American Bakers Association
- The US Potato Board
- The American Italian Pasta Company

The ADA's comments were a series of extremely brief recommendations filed jointly in every single instance with the American Heart Association and the American Cancer Society. Apparently not one independent word needed to be said about the unique nature of type 2 diabetes, the only disease of the three with a clear-cut dietary origin. "Diabetes? Cancer? Hey, what's the difference, anyway?" seemed to be the attitude.

I asked the ADA about the lack of dietary differentiation. Here's what they had to say:

"We worked together [with those two organizations] to respond because two out of three deaths in the United States are due to cancer, diabetes, heart disease and stroke. The bottom line is that these diseases are largely preventable through healthy diets, physical activity and maintenance of a healthy weight. We see the value in collaborating with other organizations to raise the visibility and awareness of disease prevention and health promotion and felt that our combined statement would have a greater impact than working in isolation."

My take: True, those diseases cause two in three deaths, but that's like combining the leading causes of accidental deaths simply because they add up to a big percentage—and then offering exactly the same advice for preventing both drownings and car wrecks. As for exercise and diet preventing the vast majority of cases, to suggest that dietary decisions can ward off cancer at any level comparable to diabetes— which is, after all, a direct and entirely predictable result of unhealthy eating—is specious. And collaborating for collaboration's sake is more important than offering diabetes-specific information to the dietary guidelines committee? You've already read the roster of carb promoters who chimed in. The USDA probably would have made note of what the ADA had to say about sugar, seeing as how they're the main diabetes organization. The problem is that they seem to have nothing unique to say about it.

No matter what dietary regime one believes is best for combating type 2 diabetes, there's no way that perfunctory, joint input is sufficient for preventing and managing this disease.

TO UNDERSTAND THE ADA's current dietary guidance, you need to understand its evolution. "Forty or fifty years ago, their guidelines were more opinion documents than something designed to be followed by a broad slew of people," says Dr. Gale, the Bristol University diabetes professor. "Now, very self-consciously, the ADA sees itself as the source of authoritative information on every aspect of diabetes. Therefore, the ADA expects to have a regularly updated view on everything. They don't necessarily expect that to represent the final word of scientific opinion, but they do expect it to represent good, sensible advice that the physician or patient can follow without coming to harm."

The question is how sensible that advice has been. "The ADA completely missed the boat on managing sugar and insulin," says nutrition expert and author Jonny Bowden. Isn't that sort of like the American Cancer Society missing the boat on the perils of cigarette smoking? Could anyone reasonably say: "People will smoke regardless, so let's accept that and make *the focus* of our public-health effort the long-term management of lung cancer?" No. The official lifestyle guidelines of the

American Cancer Society start by calling for smoking cessation because therein lies the solution.

The ADA has published three major position statements on nutrition in *Diabetes Care*, one of its official journals, over the past two decades. The 1994 nutrition guidelines didn't exactly revise the 1986 macronutrient architecture of 60 percent carb, less than 30 percent fat, and the rest from protein. What they did was leave protein at 10 percent, make saturated fat less than 10 percent of calories, and leave the rest to a patient's discretion, based on "nutrition assessment and treatment goals." Given that many doctors know so little about the intersection of diet and diabetes, what are they supposed to be assessing? As for treatment goals, what is there besides (a) avoiding diabetes or (b) delaying its progression once you have it? If I had been prediabetic back in 1994, that scheme would have told me nothing that I needed to know about fighting the disease.

The 2002 guidelines were similarly obscure and nonspecific, aside from minor tinkering with the protein range. Nothing suggested that the ADA was distancing itself from the low-fat mantra of the past, however. On the contrary, "For weight loss, dietary fat is probably the most important nutrient to be restricted," the authors wrote. We've already seen how that played out over the three decades leading up to those guidelines: dietary fat, down 3 to 4 percent; obesity, up 16 percent—hardly an Rx for type 2 diabetes.

The 2008 guidelines actually gave a grudging nod to carb cutting, but only for short-term weight loss. They reflected no change in the basic carb prescription for diabetics, that is, how many should be consumed or avoided to tame this metabolic beast. Often the language is so vague that it's hard to tell what the ADA thinks, exactly, about carbs and fat at this point.

In an e-mail exchange with me, the ADA summed up its current take on carbs: "We continue to emphasize that individuals with diabetes should have a personalized approach to managing their diabetes that meets their goals for weight management, blood glucose, blood lipids, and blood pressure. We do not set a minimum or maximum amount of carbohydrate that people with diabetes should eat to manage their diabetes and there is nothing [to that effect] in our guidelines."

No guidelines means no dietary restrictions. And isn't that a big part of the problem?

"THEY WOULD NEVER say, 'Oh, we were wrong,' but they seem to be quietly backing away from their advice that you should eat a low-fat, high-carb diet," says Stanford's Dr. Reaven.

Many critics of the decades-running higher-carb approach found this nascent shift—if indeed it even is a shift; who can tell?—overdue and tepid. Instead of leading us in the wrong direction, the ADA guidelines are now leading us around in circles. They're essentially telling us that the diet that's healthy for someone with diabetes is no different from the diet that's healthy for everyone else, with appropriate calorie restrictions for the overweight. When I asked the ADA if that is indeed the case, they responded, "It is often generalized that a diet that is healthy for people with diabetes, is good for the whole family."

The problem with this is twofold. First, the diet that's supposed to be good for everyone is making the majority of people overweight, which in turn raises their odds of becoming diabetic. The second is best expressed through a simple logic exercise: The metabolism of Mr. Jones can handle carbs properly. The metabolism of Mr. Smith, the diabetic or prediabetic, treats carbs as if they were poison. That's *why* he's diabetic. Yet he should eat the same amount of carbs? How can that possibly be sound advice?

Aside from that recent nod to a lower-carb approach for short-term weight loss only, the guidelines don't contain the sort of concrete recommendation that will change the way doctors discuss type 2 diabetes with their patients. With obesity and diabetes ballooning, we need more than a little fine-tuning here.

THE TERM "LOW-CARB diet" is bandied about all the time, but what does it mean, really? Dietary recommendations encourage Americans to consume 45 to 65 percent of all calories in the form of carbs, so any alternative approach whose carb allocation falls below 45 percent could be deemed a low-carb diet, or at least a lower-carb diet.

As a concept, "low carb" could also be applied to any dietary regimen where someone deliberately restricts their carb intake, or consciously chooses carbs with a low glycemic index or load, instead of eating whatever looks yummy. A low-carb devotee would typically account for both dietary concerns: the total amount of carbs *and* their glycemic effects. Both of these things would matter. They do to me.

But "low-carb diet" has more rigorous connotations for dietitians, nutritionists, and even the public at large, courtesy of books such as *Dr. Atkins' New Diet Revolution* and *The South Beach Diet*. Americans hungry for answers to their weight problem have purchased many millions of copies of these volumes.

I like this breakdown, which I read in a nutrition journal:

• The authors defined a "low-carbohydrate ketogenic diet" as less than 50 grams of carbs a day (less than 10 percent of total calories). Here, your body burns so much fat for fuel that it makes ketones. An even more restrictive version—the Atkins "induction" phase, with its 20-gram cutoff—amounts to a nutritional war against dietary carbs. If you think of diabetes as a metabolic fire, imagine the oxygen being cut off. Turning it off is one thing; keeping it off requires real discipline.

• A "low-carbohydrate diet" was defined in the table as 50 to 130 grams of carbs a day (10 to 26 percent of total calories, respectively, if someone's eating 2,000 calories a day).

• A "moderate-carbohydrate diet" was defined as 130 to 225 grams of carbs a day, or 26 to 45 percent of total calories.

These gaps are wide. Even if you compare a midrange low-carb figure (say, 20 percent of calories) with the "normal" mean (55 percent) of the dietary recommendations for average Americans, the difference is 35 percent. No matter what your opinion is in this debate, for better or worse your body will look and feel much, much different at 20 percent carbs than it will at 55 percent.

One of the keys to reducing type 2 diabetes is reducing obesity, and studies have proven what people already knew from experience: Cut the carbs, melt the body fat. The losses are quicker and more pronounced than on diets where carbs aren't squeezed. Why do low-carb dieters lose weight so fast? "When people reduce their carbs, they just eat less," says Braun, the exercise-as-medicine expert. "All these high-carb snack foods are suddenly off-limits, and they don't replace them." The research backs this up.

"Once you get the physiology right, patient behavior changes," Dr. Westman says of patients at his weight-loss clinic, noting protein and fat turn off the brain's hunger signal, but carbs don't. Cut the carbs, and—ta-da!—dieters have willpower.

You won't need to eat as much, assuming you burn roughly the same number of calories. Your body won't need to produce as many triglycerides, which it had been cranking out because it had to do something with all that glucose that wasn't being properly disposed of. Since your muscle cells are no longer hungry, your appetite will diminish as well.

The results will be visible. If you're like Ian McIntyre, a sixty-four-year-old former small-business consultant, you might be wearing a belt with an extra notch punched into it—by hand. The belt I'm looking at in Dr. Westman's examination room is the second one McIntyre's had to mutilate because the flaps became ridiculously long. That's fine by him. When he arrived at the clinic, the Durham resident was a 289-pound diabetic with a fasting blood glucose reading of 170 mg/dL, well past the diabetes cutoff point of 126. After cutting out the carbs, per doctor's orders, McIntyre has seen his weight fall to 238, en route to 190. "I *will* get there," he tells me.

Unlike other diets that he has tried off and on for years, this one doesn't require dietary deprivation. "There's no hunger going on," says McIntyre, now in retirement. "That's the beauty of it, and that's why I knew I could stick with it almost from the start." His appetite is under control. The blood sugar fluctuations that cause people to fall off other diets are smoothed out here. Stick with the diet like Ian did and those fat stores will shrink, along with your waistline. At that point, fat cells will no longer be able to draw from their reserves to replace the missing carb calories. After a while, hunger will kick in. Carb cutters often trip up here. "They understand that they're to avoid carbs, but they've been indoctrinated to avoid fat as well," says Dr. Wortman. When hunger beckons, don't give in and reach for the sweets. Feed your body protein instead.

Neither man nor woman can live happily on turkey and tofu alone, however. Some popular low-carb diets attempt to solve this problem by gently bumping up the carbs until hunger becomes less of a nag. Not so fast, says Dr. Wortman: "Increased carbs drives increased appetite, making you eat more and more of the inappropriate carbohydrate, leading to weight gain."

Having used up its own blubber, the body will take dietary fat and start burning its by-products, called fatty acids or ketones, for energy. That's why a person can eat more fat without becoming fatter. What's more, as insulin resistance weakens, energy floods into cells. The signals to eat up and reserve energy are reversed; if you eat fat the signal now becomes, "Gee, get up and run around! You have lots of energy now. Oh, and by the way, stop eating so much!"

So as it turns out, you are *not* what you eat. Instead you are what you *do* with what you eat. Carb control makes the human body a fat-burning machine. "Switching metabolism from carbs to a fat fuel source is a very powerful tool once you learn how to use it," says Volek. Like Dr. Westman, he eats as if he's allergic to carbs, even though he looks lean and fit, sitting across a conference table from me at the University of Connecticut. "It works great for most people, but especially for diabetics. They do very well on it."

The shift to burning fat also spares protein. This is important because during weight loss, protein spares muscle tissue. Muscle is the most metabolically active tissue, allowing for continuous fat burning, not just during workouts. Use it to your advantage.

This metabolic shift doesn't happen overnight, but almost. During my first cold, dark winter of carb-controlled living in Pennsylvania as a man on the verge of diabetes, I wondered where this was leading me, and how I would feel once I arrived. Initially I felt as if hunger was my constant companion. Sugar had come to rule my body, and it was anything but a benevolent dictator. Now I was suffering withdrawal pangs. I found myself thinking about food all the time.

Fortunately the hunger between meals didn't last long. I felt the shift happening within weeks. Soon enough, my body normalized. The shadow vanished.

Within a matter of months, my weight had fallen from 220 pounds to 195. Today the needle is pegged at 185. I've come to believe that when I eat the way I'm supposed to eat, my body just weighs what it's supposed to weigh. Period. The deviation is no more than two or three pounds up or down. My scale wound up in the same place as those meds for high blood pressure—in the trash.

Dr. Westman's patients come to his clinic to shed pounds, but they leave with a bonus. The diabetes they often have seems to vanish with the excess baggage. Obesity and diabetes tend to be caused by the same thing, insulin resistance. Dr. Westman's carb-avoidance program cures both ills at once.

"There is no better way to control glucose," says Dr. Westman. The need for diabetes meds goes away fast. Based on clinical experience, he now reduces a patient's insulin *before* the first carb has even been cut. Otherwise patients will risk going too low too fast.

But is the weight loss produced by low-carb dieting the *only* reason these diets improve glucose metabolism in patients such as Ian McIntyre? If so, the same benefits could theoretically be derived from severe caloric restriction, or any other effective weight-loss regimen.

At the Metabolic Research Laboratory at the VA Medical Center in Minneapolis, a pair of University of Minnesota diabetes researchers wanted to tease out the effects of a low-carb diet on blood glucose, apart from any loss of body weight. Mary C. Gannon, Ph.D., professor of food science and nutrition at the University of Minnesota, and her research partner Frank Q. Nuttall, M.D., Ph.D., designed what they call Low Biologically Available Glucose (LoBAG) diets. During the study, caloric management kept subjects at the same weight for the whole experiment.

Those on the LoBAG diets showed significant improvements in all

their metabolic markers. The lower the carbs, the better the results, which sort of makes you wonder why she doesn't lower them even more. By the time subjects were down to 20 or 30 percent carbs, their blood glucose had fallen almost 40 percent. Moreover their fasting glucose measurements approached normal. "Altering the diet composition could be a patient-empowering method of improving the hyperglycemia of type 2 diabetes without weight loss or pharmacologic intervention," wrote the researchers.

Rather than being the original catalyst, weight loss is another positive response to carb restriction. A greater improvement in glucose metabolism comes from losing weight on low carbs than from losing it another way. That's a double dose of good news. You can still achieve major metabolic improvements with or without weight loss.

Carb-restricted diets can have other positive effects on cardiovascular health. Within six months to two years, the risk factors for having a heart attack can significantly decrease. In another weight-loss trial, this one spanning twenty-four weeks, a low-carb diet outperformed a low-fat diet at lowering triglycerides and raising HDL, the healthy cholesterol. The low-carb group also shed more pounds. Not bad for people turning conventional wisdom on its head by eating more saturated fat and cholesterol but fewer carbs than they were before.

ONE STOCK ARGUMENT against carb restriction, even for diabetics, is that people don't stay the course. Sure, they lose some weight after they cut carbs, but often they stumble and gain it right back, the argument goes. Of course, this could be said of any diet. Low-carb diets won't work without adherence, just as low-fat diets certainly won't work if the person starts eating three times a day at Burger King.

Losing weight is not easy. But if someone is going to make the effort, they should at least be using the approach that will reward adherence with results. For diabetics, that approach is carb reduction.

If you think you're too busy to watch calories and carbs, spend a day in the company of Dr. Vernon. The 58-year-old is a force of nature,

reminding me of a midwestern version of Dame Judi Dench, with a tousled, Q-like haircut to match. Trying to follow her intellectual dexterity in conversation, I feel like the pursuer in a car chase. As it turns out, the low-carb diet she recommends to patients is what keeps those brain circuits humming. "One of the reasons I eat this way," she says over lunch at an Italian restaurant in Lawrence, "is that my output is so high." She smiles. "I can do lots of stuff."

I've been accused (incorrectly) of being a workaholic, but listening to her, I think I must be a real slacker. Besides being a family practice physician carrying a patient load that would bury most doctors, she works in a local ER several nights a week, holds high positions in several national metabolic societies, writes books and journal articles, and runs what amounts to an animal rescue from the home she shares with her partner, Sarah. She has a son from a prior marriage, so add motherhood to the list.

Inside Dr. Vernon's clinic, I meet many patients from all walks of life and of all body types. A 38-year-old woman named Tracy Claycamp reminds me of me. She's thin and healthy . . . *looking*, but she, too, has insulin resistance, metabolic obesity, and a red-flagged medical history: her mother's liver developed cirrhosis. Tracy, a cardiac nurse, wondered why a woman who never drank was now on the waiting list for a transplant. Then there was her own fatigue. *Okay, maybe that's just how any young mother feels*, she thought. But how to explain her constant hunger, despite eating?

Insulin resistance can lead to nonalcoholic fatty liver disease before diabetes. When Dr. Vernon tested Tracy, her insulin was thirteen times normal. Hence the fatigue and hunger. "If I had continued down that path, I probably would have ended up in the same situation that my mom is in," says Tracy, a young son bouncing around her knees.

She took ownership of her situation by eliminating sugars from her diet three years ago. She loves eating this way and wouldn't consider lapsing. Why would she? She feels great and is shielded from her mom's fate. That's the best compliance strategy there is—giving patients tools that work. What a novel concept, as opposed to rattling off reason after reason why patients will fail in the end.

I mention to Dr. Vernon how her patients all seem so engaged in their treatment. They discuss their illness with their doctor, ask insightful, challenging questions, and become data driven, analyzing their own blood work results. *This is how it should work,* I thought to myself. There's nothing special about these people. They represent a random sample from a college town in the heartland. This could happen anywhere. If we reimagine our approach to preventing and treating type 2 diabetes, it could happen everywhere.

A common criticism of low-carb eating is that those highly prone to type 2 diabetes, the poor, give up quickly. Tell that to another of Dr. Vernon's patients, Daniel L. Hayes. This 70-year-old semiretiree bakes and washes dishes at the local Perkins three nights a week. He came to her as an obese, type 2 diabetic taking a blood sugar medication called glyburide.

She put him on a low-carb diet, told him to junk the meds.

"I lost several pounds with Dr. Vernon's—" he says in a slow southern drawl.

"Several would be like fifty," she chimes in.

"Eighty," he says, laughing. "I went from 248 to 172 pounds in fourteen months on her diet. And my blood glucose went from, what, 260, I believe it was, down to 123. The VA decided I wasn't diabetic enough anymore to warrant paying for my test strips."

The VA also had to throw him out of a hypertension study he was enrolled in, as his blood pressure returned to normal on the diet.

"So I guess he's not sick anymore," she says, laughing at the absurdity. "That must be what it means, right, if they won't give you the testing supplies anymore?"

What it means is that our health care system rewards failure and penalizes success when it comes to diabetes. Of course he should keep monitoring his blood sugar! Self-empowerment has been part of his cure. Why on earth would you take away this guy's positive reinforcement, now that he's winning?

If a guy who bakes pies at Perkins can stick to a low-carb diet, anyone can.

The son of a child psychiatrist, Dr. Westman has success teaching a low-carb diet even to those living on food stamps. They've come to one of his two Duke University clinics hoping to lose weight, and he's snatched away all of their refined sugar and flour, the cheap energy sources that have fueled them their whole lives. He's taking comfort foods away from people who desperately need comfort. And yet it works, in part because he spends the necessary time explaining *why* he wants them to change their diet.

He makes it simple. He hands them a list of foods and says, "If you only eat from this list, this will work." A permissible snack that North Carolinians seem particularly fond of is crunchy pork skins slathered with pimento cheese, which sounds like it would go well with *Monday Night Football*. Believe it or not, there are no rules or even guidance for portion size. Self-regulation works where enforcement didn't. Once their physiology has been fixed, patients instinctively reduce the amount they eat.

At a Mexican restaurant near his clinic, Dr. Westman orders fajitas and spurns the flour tortilla and rice for lunch. The doctor doesn't seem to have an ounce of fat on his body, and his blood sugar and insulin are as synchronized as a Rolex. Still, he practices what he preaches. "Excellent nutrition, tasty foods, and appetite suppression," he tells me when I ask why. He points to research showing that a diet without sugar and starch is healthier than a diet with them.

That contradicts another tired critique of the low-carb approach. Avoid diabetes on low carbs, they say, and a heart attack will get you. Maybe not. Once the body has shifted to fat burning, it begins handling saturated fat differently. One study found that while low-carb dieters ingested three times more saturated fat than they did before enrolling, measures of saturated fat in their blood went down, not up. When carbs are low and insulin isn't stimulating much fat synthesis, the body can burn more saturated fat for fuel.

Fat's fate rests with carbs. One common mistake to avoid when consuming more fat is to then reintroduce the carbs. Even small rises in insulin downshift the body's ability to burn fat. Under this scenario, saturated fat might be dealt with in a more harmful way. Consider it one more reason to avoid junk food, which is high in both carbs and fat.

Another critique of the low-carb approach is a lack of long-term research. Unfortunately for patients who are sick now, and becoming sicker by the day, the research on low-carb dieting and diabetes is a good decade behind the clinical experience, according to Dr. Westman. Indeed many of the low-carb studies have been shorter term and with smaller sample sizes—all the more reason to get moving on longer-term research. ADA told me that of the approximately four thousand research projects they've funded, about twenty-six have focused on carbohydrates since 1970.

I'd be curious to know if slightly more than one-half of 1 percent of the American Cancer Society's research has focused on smoking cessation.

10

SWEET SURRENDER

When most of us think of sugar, we picture a spoonful of white crystals. You might assume that inserting said spoon into your mouth would be the quickest way to antagonize your blood sugar. Actually, no. That white stuff is called sucrose, and the chemical composition is half fructose, half glucose. Only the glucose half is pure sugar. Nevertheless table sugar is still deemed a "simple" carb, meaning that digestive enzymes can take them apart with ease, and they flood the bloodstream.

Other carbs, called starches, comprise long strands of glucose molecules—simple sugars—bound together to form what are called polysaccharides, or "complex" carbs. As soon as saliva meets starch, those chemical bonds begin disintegrating. Sometimes, however, that process takes longer than breaking down simple sugars.

But not always. Eat a baked potato, and pure sugar (glucose) hits your bloodstream in a heartbeat. This complex carb doesn't stay complex for very long after you eat it; a baked potato can spike blood sugar faster than eating a spoonful of table sugar. That's why the typical rec-ommendation for diabetics to consume carbs, just so long as they are "complex," is misleading in many respects.

When my father was my age, people played Russian roulette with their blood sugar any time they consumed carbs; no one even thought about it. Today, however, thanks to the glycemic index, a person can know in advance what effect a particular carb will have on the glucose coursing through his or her veins. Developed in the early 1980s, the glycemic index rates carbs based on their transit speed, which is the time needed for carbs to move from the stomach to the bloodstream. This tells you how they'll affect your blood sugar. The scale goes from 0 to 100, and foods and beverages are given numbers that mean they're high, medium, or low glycemic. The lower the number, the more slowly that carb breaks down in the body. And the slower, the better. For example:

High Glycemic (70 or Above)
    Dates: 103
    Rice Chex: 89
    Baked potato: 85
    Cornflakes: 83
    Pretzels: 81
    Jelly beans: 80
    Gatorade: 78
    Potato chips: 75
    Corn chips: 74
    Pop Tarts: 70

Medium Glycemic (56 to 69)
    Froot Loops: 69
    Shredded Wheat: 69
    Raisins: 64
    White rice: 58
    Fruit cocktail: 55
    Popcorn: 55

Low Glycemic (55 or Below)
> Bananas: 54
>
> Oranges: 44
>
> Chickpeas: 33
>
> Chocolate milk: 24
>
> Artichoke, asparagus, broccoli, cauliflower, celery, cucumber, eggplant, green beans, lettuce, peppers, spinach, tomatoes, and zucchini: all 15

These are estimates, since every human body is unique. Your blood sugar might react differently to a banana than mine, and a person's *own* glycemic response to a given carb can vary 25 to 50 percent from one measure to the next, depending on a number of factors. A carb's glycemic index remains roughly the same, aside from minor changes caused by method of preparation, ripeness, and so on, but your insulin sensitivity will fluctuate in response to everything, from natural body rhythms to a workout or a prior meal. If different carbs also were tested at those same moments, theoretically, the same variation should apply.

Despite these variations, the glycemic index offers an educated estimate of how a given carb will interact with your blood sugar relative to other carbs. This matters because the blood glucose concentration from a high-glycemic food is at least twice that of a low-glycemic within two hours of consumption. The pancreas needs to supply a commensurate amount of insulin. Insulin signals the body to store fat. So high-glycemic carbs unleash a chain of events leading to belly flab, especially since the insulin-induced blood-sugar crash stokes hunger for more carbs. In a study published in the *Journal of the American Medical Association*, obese teenagers fed a high-glycemic-index breakfast consumed 600 to 700 more calories at lunch than teens starting their day with a low-glycemic-index breakfast.

Studies have also linked a low-glycemic-index diet to a reduced risk for type 2 diabetes, cardiovascular disease, and cancer, although certainly the weight-loss benefits may be contributing to all three of these beneficial outcomes.

The glycemic index is helpful, but it doesn't account for the *quantity* of carbs contained in foods. An apple might contain high-glycemic-index carbs, but it doesn't contain nearly as many of those fast-acting carbs as a glass of apple juice, where the fiber has been processed out. So another measure, glycemic load, divides the GI by 100 and then multiplies that sum by the number of carbs (excluding fiber, sugar alcohols, and other carbs that can't be readily digested) contained in a food. Watermelon, for example, contains fast-acting carbs as measured by the glycemic index, but it has a low glycemic load because of the water content. Then again, some foods containing slower carbs are so densely packed with them that they pile up fast. Oatmeal and couscous fall in this category. They're very solid carb choices for diabetics, but the glycemic load warns that they can be easily overeaten, unlike, say, broccoli and tomatoes. If I have a vegetable omelet, coffee, and water for breakfast, I might ask for a cup of oatmeal on the side, with no milk or brown sugar added. For the rest of the day, most of my carbs will come from nonstarchy vegetables and a little fruit.

As a result, the glycemic load concept may be even more useful than the glycemic index for diabetics, although the key number is still total number of carbs, minus fiber. The glycemic index and load are only starting points for carb management, but they beat the heck out of flying blind. In 1998, two United Nations agencies, the World Health Organization and the Food and Agriculture Organization, endorsed the glycemic index as useful for treating both obesity and type 2 diabetes. Unfortunately, they also upped their carb recommendations.

The ADA was more muted about the index when it released a new position statement on nutrition and diabetes four years later, in 2002. "Although it is clear that carbohydrates do have differing glycemic responses, the data reveal no clear trend in outcome benefits. If there are long-term effects on glycemia and lipids, these effects appear to be modest," the authors wrote. That stance was reiterated in a 2004 update of those recommendations.

In another change to be filed under the heading BETTER LATE THAN NEVER, the ADA refined its position on the glycemic index when it released its next major position statement on nutrition and diabetes, in 2008. "The use of glycemic index and load may provide a modest additional benefit over that observed when total carbohydrate is considered alone," wrote the authors in the section on managing diabetes. Hardly a ringing endorsement that was. The section on preventing diabetes, as opposed to managing it, suggested that insufficient evidence exists at present to conclude that low-glycemic-load diets reduce diabetes risk. Oddly, they don't mention low-glycemic-*index* diets.

A 2008 review published on low-glycemic-index diets and diabetes took an exhaustive tour through the research, much as the ADA must have done as part of writing up their evidence-based guidelines. I found myself wondering just how much evidence is required before a recommendation is made. This review looked at retrospective, epidemiological, and pilot studies; randomized control trials; and studies of studies, called meta-analyses. The vast majority found statistically significant benefits to glucose metabolism, blood sugar levels, or both from lowering a diet's glycemic index.

According to many of the experts with whom I spoke, a trickle of the wrong carbs is preferable to an avalanche of the better ones. Sure, whole wheat bread falls lower on the glycemic index than white bread. Yet both products break down into sugar in the end. The same goes for brown rice versus white rice. With a glycemic index 10 points lower than white rice, carbs from brown rice enter the bloodstream more slowly. But they still arrive. Is brown rice better than white for diabetics? Surely. But that switch alone doesn't even begin to address the problem.

The glycemic index is an easy-to-understand tool that allows diabetics to differentiate among a bewildering array of daily carb choices. Without it, under the American Dietetic Association's guidelines, diabetics could theoretically be consuming 65 percent of their calories from carbs such as mashed potatoes, croissants, white bread, Rice Krispies, and straight glucose—all of which have a glycemic index of 70 or above. As someone on the cusp of type 2 diabetes, considering how my blood sugar is affected by different carbs, as measured by the glycemic index and load, seems like a no-brainer. If I want to live a long, full, healthy life, how could I *not* be mindful of such a fundamental blood sugar consideration?

I'm not arguing in favor of emblazoning glycemic index and load data on all food labels, as some people suggest. Such labeling risks creating the same trap that formed during the low-fat craze. Consumers might see "low glycemic" and believe they can eat to their heart's desire with impunity. But the official guidelines should argue more persuasively for doctors to educate patients about the glycemic effects of various carbs.

Of course, the lower the number of carbs consumed, the less need to obsess about where those carbs fall on any chart. "The main game is the amount of carbohydrate in your diet," says Raab. "That's what sends blood sugar shooting straight up." And only bad things happen from there, whether blood sugar stays high or comes crashing back down.

CERTAIN FOODS ARE craved precisely because they contain so much energy in so little volume. To feed the addiction, we're mainlining sugar in progressively larger doses. That's part of the problem. The other part of the problem—the real problem, some might say—is the degree to which food-processing technology concentrates sugar, and the energy density of foods as a result. The sweet science goes back to those Indian scientists who first crystallized sugar. The most recent game changer was the discovery by Japanese food scientists, made in the 1960s, that cornstarch could be turned into a clear, sweet goop called high-fructose corn syrup. Producers now had something sweeter and cheaper than cane sugar, and with a shelf life that could be measured in presidential administrations.

HFCS and soft drinks were a perfect match, but not the only one. HFCS found its way into nearly everything we eat and drink. Ketchup, crackers, cereal, yogurt, baked goods, salad dressing, condiments, and seemingly everything else on supermarket shelves contain it. The first ingredient in low-fat mayonnaise? HFCS. During the two decades leading up to 1990, HFCS consumption in the United States increased tenfold. By 1999, average HFCS consumption topped out at a whopping 215 calories' worth per person per day.

Fructose doesn't have the sudden, dramatic effect on blood sugar that glucose does, but it presents issues of its own. It produces what are called advanced glycation end products ("AGE") at a rate ten times greater than that triggered by glucose. Normally only a small fraction of your bloodstream's sugar content becomes glycated; the rest is used for metabolism. But in diabetics with chronic hyperglycemia, AGE formation accelerates to a dangerous rate. The body can handle these rogue agents, but only slowly, since AGEs stick around twice as long as average cells. Especially prone are long-lived cells such as nerve cells, collagen proteins, and DNA; and metabolically active cells, which happens to include cells in the pancreas (beta), kidneys, and retina. Weakening of the collagen in blood-vessel walls leads to hypertension and heightens stroke risk. And fructose increases the oxidation of LDL particles, raising the specter of heart disease.

You wouldn't know that from those commercials. Maybe you've seen them. In one, a pretty Caucasian mom at what appears to be a children's birthday party approaches a pretty African American mom. The latter is pouring a cupful of something that looks like red antifreeze, prompting the first mom to grimace. She says, "You don't care what the kids eat, huh? . . . You know what they say about high-fructose corn syrup."

"Like what?" asks the mom pouring the red swill, looking like the cat that swallowed the canary. "That it's made from corn, doesn't have artificial ingredients, and, like sugar, is fine in moderation?"

Score one for the makers of HFCS? Well, it's easy to win an argument when you're filming the commercial.

The debate is more complicated than saying, "HFCS is made from corn, which is a vegetable—so, hey, it's good for you!" as the corn lobby insists. The point isn't: "Hey, this stuff is no worse than sucrose." Rather, it's: "Hey, this stuff is just as bad as sucrose." Pick your metabolic poison.

I've heard a number of HFCS critics who claim the sweetener affects the body in ways much different from and worse than sucrose, that it has uniquely harmful effects on glucose metabolism, insulin secretion, triglycerides, and abdominal fat. Most of these "HFCS-is-the-devil's-candy" claims are still being argued, and I don't find many of them all that compelling, at least when it comes to differentiating HFCS from sucrose *as ingredients*.

Having said that, all the HFCS-bashing does reinforce the idea that all concentrated forms of sugar (HFCS, sucrose, dextrose, organic cane juice, and numerous others found in sweeteners and syrups) are harmful when they total twenty-two teaspoons of added sugar a day, the amount now consumed by John and Jane Q. Public. That's sixteen and thirteen more teaspoons than men and women, respectively, should be consuming daily, according to a recent American Heart Association scientific statement. Imagine what that adds up to over a month, over a year, over a lifetime—a lifetime that probably isn't going to be as long as it should be with such high sugar consumption.

As the University of Washington's Drewnowski points out, the real problem is that sugar calories are cheap, and lower-income families, especially, consume way too many of them in solid forms such as sweetened cereals, semisolid forms such as smoothies, semiliquid forms such as yogurt, *and* liquid forms such as soda. HFCS just happens to account for 40 percent of the market for substitute sugars, excluding calorie-free ones such as Equal and Splenda.

How did it take over? "Just when America was beginning to understand that too much sugar is bad, the perception developed that fructose was okay because it didn't impact blood sugar so much," nutrition commentator Jonny Bowden told me. "HFCS didn't have the bad PR, plus it was cheaper. That, plus a pro-corn agriculture policy, made it the perfect alternative to sugar for food manufacturers. Even though it isn't all that different from plain old sugar, the fact that it was so much sweeter and cheaper led to its addition to hundreds of products that didn't contain sugar before, such as salad dressings and hamburger buns. HFCS became ubiquitous and led to a meteoric rise in overall sugar consumption. We may have been consuming (virtually identical) sucrose before the late 1960s, but we weren't consuming nearly as much because it wasn't as accessible as HFCS."

In the United States, two-thirds of all HFCS consumption comes in liquid form. A twelve-ounce soda contains the equivalent of eight teaspoons of sugar. This helps explain how people could be consuming those twenty-two added teaspoons, an amount that would be sickening if eaten by the spoonful instead of blended into products by food scientists. Sweet soda has been a Trojan horse for type 2 diabetes. When Yale University researchers tracked the diets of more than 91,000 people for eight years, they found that drinkers of more than one daily soft drink were twice as likely to develop diabetes as drinkers of only one. No link was found between diabetes and sugar-free diet sodas.

The bottom line is this: Many people think HFCS is bad but that other kinds of sugar aren't. In truth, when you're diabetic, no sugar is good sugar.

WITHIN A WEEK of receiving my own diabetes wake-up call, I found myself in a supermarket in rural Pennsylvania. This was terra incognita, since I don't cook, perhaps the only lifestyle trait I share with Angelina Jolie and Katie Holmes, not to mention about half the U.S. population, according to the Bureau of Labor Statistics. It was when wandering the aisles that I realized how nearly impossible it is to avoid sugar—and how few grams of carbs 20 truly is. I was going to start with that stingy number, the amount allowed during the Atkins "induction phase," and slowly build back up from there. I viewed it as a twist on the elimination diets recommended for people with food allergies—only my allergy was to carbohydrates. Eliminate items to see if the problem improves, and if it does, add them back until the problem recurs. Those are your limits.

The contents filling most shelves were off-limits to me; they might as well have been cordoned off with police tape. Ten minutes into the excursion, as I passed a soccer mom piling boxes of sugary cereals into her overflowing cart, I glanced down at my own. It contained a copy of the new GQ, shaving cream—and cinnamon? Indeed. Another nutritionist friend of mine, Christopher Mohr, Ph.D., R.D., had told me about research suggesting that this spice helps control blood sugar. The active ingredient in this spice, a compound called hydroxychalcone, seems to improve insulin sensitivity. Jonny Bowden agreed with Mohr's advice. "Sprinkle it on everything you can," he said, although the typical daily dose is 1 gram, or half a teaspoon. "The cheap supermarket stuff works just as well as the expensive supplement versions."

There's a reason this stuff was prized medicinally by everyone from the ancient Egyptians to the Romans, who valued cinnamon more highly than gold. Still, I don't take anyone's view as gospel without my own investigation. Nor should you. The research on cinnamon and blood sugar is compelling but equivocal. A pair of studies found promising results, reductions in blood glucose levels of 20 percent or so. But other studies of cinnamon and blood sugar produced results that were wishy-washy. Nonetheless, it's a simple, inexpensive trick that, unlike diabetes drugs, does no harm, barring an allergy to the spice.

Just in case cinnamon works as advertised, I began sprinkling it into protein shakes, on cottage cheese with blueberries, even on my Chilean-style eggs. Try it; it's yummy. I'll use the spice until I read otherwise. If it turns out to be ineffective, fine. Cinnamon isn't a stand-alone diabetes treatment, and I'm confident that the dozens of other things I'm doing will rule the day. That's important to remember. Don't look at a headline about cinnamon and then think you're managing the disease simply by taking a few capsules of it a day. Without diet and exercise doing the heavy lifting, trying to control diabetes with cinnamon is like trying to extinguish a forest fire with a squirt gun.

Even worse is thinking that adding cinnamon to unhealthy items makes them okay. The cinnamon chips in Bob Evans's Cinnamon Cream Stacked & Stuffed Hotcakes don't offset the metabolic and arterial damage done by the 1,380 calories, most of them carbs, and 34 grams of saturated fat. Not even close. Or consider the Cinnabon, arguably the unhealthiest food on earth. Suffice it to say that any positive effects from cinnamon are offset many, many times over by the 117 carb grams and 32 fat grams.

I was shocked to see how the 20-gram Atkins prescription stacked up against the sort of foods I might have reached for before my blood sugar went bananas—which were now off-limits. One cup of cornflakes contains 24 grams of carbs, so that alone would exceed my new daily limit, not counting the added milk. One hot dog roll contains 26 grams.

Kraft Mac & Cheese Thick 'n Creamy weighed in at 50 grams of carbs per 2.5 ounces. Utz Sourdough Specials pretzels, the sort of snack I would have devoured while watching the Redskins play on Sunday afternoon, was good (or bad) for 21 grams of carbs per ounce.

Like many people, I seldom would eat just one of those single-serving bags—they come in 1.25-ounce sizes. Had I reached for those pretzels, I'd have torn open the family-size bag, eating half in one sitting. Those bags come in at 14 to 16 ounces, so that's about 150 grams of carbs for a snack.

If I wanted a hot dog I wouldn't stop at one, I'd have had two. And I would have washed them down with a beer, Coke, or other soda, increasing the carb count. We all do it. Eat those two hot dogs, wash them down with a Coke or two, maybe have some potato chips or some potato salad on the side, and your body needs a fire hose to pump out enough insulin to wash all that sugar from your blood into cells.

Further confusing shoppers, low-fat foods usually replace the fat with carbs. What's more, alternatives such as "whole grain," "organic," "free range," or "all-natural" this or that often don't make as big a health difference as advertised, especially for diabetics. Sometimes they're downright misleading. Dannon All Natural Yogurt sounds healthy; it even says "no artificial anything" under "all-natural." But the former is simply a trademarked marketing phrase. The product includes HFCS and modified corn starch, all part of 19 grams of sugars lurking underneath the foil.

On my first foray through the supermarket as a prediabetic shopper, I picked up a package of Barilla spaghetti. The box said it contained 42 grams of carbs, including 2 grams of fiber and 1 gram of sugar, in every 2 ounces. I set that down and picked up Barilla whole grain spaghetti. The difference was negligible: 1 fewer carb gram, 4 extra grams of fiber, and 1 more gram of sugar.

It wasn't hard to figure out that I now needed to avoid Lucky Charms and pretzels, but fake-out foods such as that whole-grain spaghetti were trying to lead me astray. The Healthy Choice Chicken Alfredo Florentine frozen entrée I was eyeing turned out to contain 31 grams of carbs. Two snacks I picked up, and put right back, were Mariani sweetened dried cranberries, at 35 carb grams per ¼ cup; and chocolate Jell-O Pudding Snacks, containing 25 carb grams per 4-ounce snack cup. Raisins contain 131 carb grams per cup, packed. Fruit-flavored, fat-free yogurt had 23.8 carb grams, all from sugars, per 4.4-ounce container.

Even Slim-Fast—a diet product, mind you—contained 18 carb grams per scoop, 30 with 8 ounces of milk added. My exasperation was complete when I reached for a bottle of Vitaminwater, only to realize that it contained 13 carb grams per 8 fluid ounces, and 32.5 grams carbs per bottle. Water!

I had swilled rivers of Coke growing up and was also on good terms with Dr Pepper and Mr. Pibb. But the rows of soda I was walking past were now off-limits except for the diet and hence sugar-free variety, which I had always hated but now would grow accustomed to drinking. That was an obvious move, but I was surprised when I picked up a carton of milk, another lifelong staple. According to the label, it had 13 grams of lactose, a sugar, per serving. Fruit juices were the real sugar shocker, though. The orange juice, apple juice, and pineapple juice I inspected contained 26, 31, and 35 grams of carbs, respectively, per fluid ounce. Smoothies and shakes? No way. Back in L. A., I'd sometimes grab a Jamba Juice for refreshment. The store's interior and marketing shtick made these drinks seem like a healthy alternative to soda. But only one of those fruity concoctions contains 137 grams of sugar, nearly double the glucose challenge presented during a metabolic stress test. An hour after finishing one, it's look out below for your blood sugar.

Beer?

Gone—at least the regular kind. I'd later discover some very-low-carb beers, such as Michelob Ultra and MGD 64, that taste surprisingly close to the real deal. Even something as healthy sounding as V8 juice—liquid vegetables, that's got to be good, right?—contains 10 grams of carbs, including 8 grams sugar, per 8 fluid ounces. You're much better off juicing fresh vegetables.

I needed foods as they appear in nature, not canned or shrink-wrapped. At the checkout, my cart was full of low-carb fruits and vegetables, cottage cheese and a block of cheddar, almonds and walnuts, and other items that would have formed a caveman's diet 30,000 years ago—or 29,950 years before type 2 diabetes became a problem. Well, maybe not the cheese. For beverages, I'd take home a six-pack of Diet Cherry Coke; ground coffee, to be drunk without sugar and milk, although cream's okay; and green tea, to be sweetened with Splenda. I'd pick up a bottle of red wine at the liquor store on the way home.

That's right, wine is an approved item on a low-carb diet, which is a good thing, since many other indulgences now would be off-limits. The carb count is about 3 grams per four-ounce glass of red, and 2 to 5 grams for the same amount of white. Even if two glasses of white merlot produce 10 grams of carbs, that still beats the 78 grams of sugar in two cans of Coke.

Drunk in moderation, wine can reduce stress. We partake of it in social settings for a very good reason. But wine is also a powerful physical relaxant. This, more than any botanical constituent, may explain why studies link a moderate amount of drinking with healthy-heart benefits specifically for diabetics. That benefit shouldn't be discounted, considering the association between diabetes and cardiovascular disease.

Wine is also one of those beverages, like coffee, that can become a surrogate for things that are much worse for your blood sugar. Lifestyle advice often loses out when it becomes too rigid and dogmatic. If you're doing everything else right, and you're having a few cups of coffee in the morning and a glass of wine with dinner, you're on the right track.

The pros outweigh the cons, of which there are a few. Alcohol is metabolized in the liver and does seem to meddle a bit with the liver's conversion of noncarb energy sources into glucose. That matters because a low-carb diet is designed to shift the fuel mix to fat and protein. This may explain why alcohol is linked more often to low blood sugar than to high. But I'd take the slight dip from a glass of wine over the spike and crash from a Jamba Juice drink. Metabolically it strikes me as being much less damaging and self-perpetuating.

IT TOOK ME only a week or two to realize that eating even small meals or snacks eight times a day as a single working professional fattens up your food bill. Bereft of kitchen skills, I gave myself permission to eat out whenever necessary, at least until I learned how to cook. But restaurants are even bigger carb minefields than supermarkets. Most menus don't break down the nutritional content of various items, and if they do, the focus is on total calories and fat grams, not on carbs. Sauces? Who knows what's lurking in those. For example, you can order something that looks healthy in print only to have it hit the table glazed with sugar.

Lunches and dinners consisting of steak or fish and fresh vegetables, or a salad overlaid with chicken, maybe dressed with oil and red-wine vinegar, or with no dressing at all, will keep you healthy. Wherever possible, I order my protein unadorned with sauce or breading, and my vegetables steamed, good choices in any Chinese restaurant. Bread isn't an option, so I ask the server to leave it in the kitchen. Temptation is a bitch.

Realizing how good these foods taste before all that junk is poured over them back in the kitchen will be a revelation. If you're like me, removing sugary treats and other junk foods from your diet will unveil the simple pleasures of natural food, perhaps for the first time in your life. Red wine paired with fresh fish and steamed broccoli can become an exquisite pleasure. Rather than feeling deprived, I began enjoying food more than I ever had before. Less became more, to paraphrase a famous architect.

In L.A. or Manhattan, carb consciousness won't raise many eyebrows, but my suddenly selective ordering elicited more than a few double takes and a bit of derision in the backwoods of eastern Pennsylvania. "Watching your girlish figure, huh?" smirked one young waitress as she snatched my menu and sauntered off.

. . .

WHEN IT COMES to insulin and blood sugar, carbs are the make-or-break macronutrient. But you have to understand the blood sugar effects of not only carbs but also protein and fat, as well as how the interactions among the three macros affect glucose metabolism. Protein foods such as eggs, turkey, and steak also affect blood sugar, in a way that's often misunderstood or overlooked. During digestion, protein's amino acids are converted into glucose—pure sugar. Theoretical models developed as far back as 1915 have suggested that a particular number of protein grams should produce half that many glucose grams in the body. At first glance, that seems like a lot of glucose for a diabetic to handle. If that were the case, a low-carb diet would be nearly as problematic a diet for diabetics as a high-carb. After all, no one wants to eat nothing but fatty foods all day.

In the 1980s, a research team did a more sophisticated, better-controlled study on the fate of glucose derived from protein. They began by feeding 50 grams of lean-beef protein to each member of a small group, some diabetic, some not. Based on the conventional wisdom, 25 grams of glucose should have been produced, enough to jolt the blood sugar of most type 2 diabetics. Instead the blood sugar of the nondiabetics was stable for four hours after consuming the beef, while the diabetics saw their glucose concentrations dip. That makes protein your staunch ally.

So what happened to those 25 grams of glucose that should have materialized? One of the study authors, Mary C. Gannon of the Lo-BAG diet fame, explained to me that nearly half (42 percent) of the protein was either used to create protein in the body, or stored as amino acids in skeletal muscle. The remainder was metabolized, but only 20 percent (not 50 percent) of the beef protein became glucose. At least part of what was left might have been stored as glycogen, she said. In study subjects, this protein-to-glucose conversion of 20 percent didn't spike blood glucose.

But why did blood sugar actually drop in the diabetics? Studies on type 2 diabetics have found that protein jump-starts insulin secretion. That may be why protein dampened the carb-induced rise in blood sugar. Eaten on their own, french fries cause a blood sugar meltdown in someone like me. But if the fries are eaten with a steak, the response is a more manageable, slower burn. That's good to know when you're seduced by the aroma of pizza and can't resist having a slice. A meat topping can actually slow the release of those carbs from the crust. Don't make pizza a habit, of course, and whatever you do, don't wash it down with soda, unless it's diet.

Unlike protein, fat by itself won't even budge your blood sugar. Nevertheless, at the ADA conference in New Orleans, Michael D. Jensen, M.D., a Mayo Clinic diabetes specialist, reviewed a series of studies, including his own, that showed that adding fat to carbs actually slows the subsequent absorption of glucose into the bloodstream. The more fat added to the meal, the greater the reduction. So if you have blood sugar problems and must eat a baked potato, put a slab of butter and bacon bits on top rather than eating it plain. Most diabetics think the opposite is true because they're told to avoid fat.

Because it's lined with nutrient-specific sensors, the stomach knows whether protein, fat, or carbs has arrived. If fat is the newcomer, those sensors will release gut hormones that exert a slow-motion effect on carbs. "Carbohydrates consumed alone are very quickly absorbed," says Sarah Berry, Ph.D., a lecturer in nutrition and dietetics at King's College London. "Including fat in the meal delays the release of nutrients from the stomach into the blood. Since glucose enters the blood more slowly, the rate of removal [by insulin] can be balanced more easily." The result: no spike, no crash, and over time, less chance of your glucose metabolism becoming impaired.

Are different types of fat more or less effective at slowing down carbs? That hasn't been thoroughly studied yet. For now, consider all fats equal for glycemic lowering, says Berry. She does suggest consuming the fat immediately before or at the same time as the carbs, rather than after them. That way, the fat has time to turn on that gut hormone response. When the carbs do hit, the feedback mechanism is already working. Remember, your glucose can be spiking within fifteen minutes of eating a gang of high-GI carbs.

When you do eat carbs, they can be "slowed down" in ways that will taste great. Here are a few suggestions:

The Carb Source (If You Must) ...	How to Slow It Down
Hamburger bun or English muffin	Dust the insides with glucomannan (see page 184 for an explanation).
Regular soda	Add a tablespoon or two of Metamucil.
Oatmeal	Add walnuts, sprinkle with cinnamon.
White rice	Eat a handful of edamame first.
Apple	Take a few bites of string cheese first.
Salad with carb items	Add avocado slices.
Chocolate	Choose the darkest you can find.
Baked potato	Top it with sour cream and bacon bits.
Pizza	Find one with a really, really thin crust and a meat topping or two.
Bread	Toast it: then butter it. Each lowers the glycemic effect.
Popcorn	Butter it.

Combining macronutrients tames your blood sugar response and makes you eat less later on. Australian researchers did a study in which participants ate energy bars that were spackled together with a bunch of sugar. The bars all had the same number of calories, but one group's bars also contained 10 grams of protein and 4 grams of fiber. At the next meal, the group whose bars contained the protein and fiber consumed almost 20 percent less sugar. No initial crash, no follow-up sugar binge.

Nuts have uniquely beneficial effects on blood sugar, especially in the presence of fast-acting carbs. Think of them as damage control if you can't stay on a strict low-carb diet. And they tend to be good choices for anyone, not just diabetics and prediabetics.

In the department of nutritional sciences at the University of Toronto, the inventors of the glycemic index, David Jenkins, Ph.D., and Cyril Kendall, Ph.D., decided to analyze the effect pistachio nuts have on the absorption of glucose into the bloodstream. Over two months, study participants fasted overnight before feeding on slices of white bread along with varying amounts (one, two, and three ounces) of pistachios. The researchers found that pistachios may help stave off heart disease and type 2 diabetes both by lessening those heart-damaging glucose leaps and insulin surges after the high-sugar carbs in white bread enter the digestive system. The results were similar whether the carbs came from potatoes, pasta, rice, or the aforementioned white bread. The more pistachios eaten, the better the glycemic control became. What's more, the blood sugar rise was negligible when the pistachios were eaten alone, making them a great diabetic snack food.

Jenkins and Kendall achieved similar results in other studies using almonds. These and other nuts contain protein, fiber, and monounsaturated fat—all of which slow the absorption of glucose into the bloodstream. Nuts also contain antioxidants, which could help offset the inflammatory response to high insulin levels. Nuts lower heart-disease risk by lowering levels of bad cholesterol, but their ability to defuse postmeal blood sugar spikes appears to be another mechanism.

Nuts have proven to be invaluable for me, given that my daily diet consists of eight small meals rather than three big ones. A handful of walnuts or almonds can become part of any meal, whether eaten like popcorn or tossed onto cottage cheese or a salad. I eat them as a dessert, too. Their monounsaturated fat and fiber turns hunger from a roar to a whimper.

Fiber is a particularly potent weapon against high blood sugar—despite being a carb, technically. In fact, it's a polysaccharide, just like those dreaded starches, the carbs that are worse than table sugar. But the sugar molecules making up fiber are bundled in such a way that our digestive systems can't break them apart. Since fiber is indigestible, the body doesn't metabolize it as it does other carbs. Fiber is neither turned into glucose nor absorbed by the bloodstream.

Better still, fiber steadies the unsettling influence nonfibrous carbs

exert on blood sugar. "Fiber decreases the absorption of anything consumed with it," says Dr. Ahmann. "If you drink a glass of apple juice,
the sugar will be absorbed quickly. However, if you eat an apple, your
body doesn't have to respond with this insulin blast." Along those same
lines, if you absolutely can't resist the occasional sugar-filled soft drink,
at least spike it with a tablespoon of Benefiber or Metamucil. This
simple trick will lower the drink's glycemic index. Your pancreas will
thank you.

Fiber also helps diabetics feel full, so they eat less. Unfortunately,
food processing tends to remove fiber. So while most people go way
overboard on added sugars, they fall well short of the 20 to 25 grams of
fiber they should consume. Even if you're cutting back on grains, fruits
and vegetables can supply most of that amount. But only if you eat the
actual fruits and vegetables rather than drinking juices based on them.

There's fiber, and then there's *fiber*. I found myself experimenting
with glucomannan, something I had read about in a fitness magazine.
Glucomannan is what's known as a water-soluble polysaccharide, which
is different from the conventional fiber additives that dissolve in water.
This stuff is so viscous that coming into contact with water expands
the powder's volume fiftyfold. If other fibers stabilize blood sugar by
slowing down the digestion and absorption of carbs, glucomannan traps
them like quicksand.

I ordered a bag online. When the package arrived, I took it for a test
drive. I added less than a single tablespoon to a glass of water, and the
white powder instantly became a gelatinous goop. To drink it, I poured
the powder into a glass of water, stirred, raised the glass to my lips, and
took several big gulps—all in a matter of seconds. A friend who contends
with blood sugar issues of her own later shared a trick. "I mix it with
my food," she told me. "It thickens up foods such as oatmeal, and my
blood sugars were awesome. I never felt so good and I was losing weight."

If you can't resist a burger with the bun, or a breakfast sandwich on
a bagel or an English muffin, give the inside of one half a light dusting
with this stuff. I do the same thing with slices of fruit. The blood-sugar,
weight-loss, and cholesterol-lowering results it produces are dramatic.
Glucomannan is the sort of simple, natural, inexpensive antidote to type

2 diabetes that nobody bothers explaining to victims of the disease, perhaps because there's no drug company foisting it upon doctors.

After being diagnosed with prediabetes, I used published research and expert interviews to guide me. One thing that became clear is that dietary supplements can be useful for diabetics and prediabetics. If you have either condition, you, like everyone, should be taking a basic multivitamin/mineral and fish oil. But that's just for starters. Find a good low- or no-carb protein powder. You should be eating small, frequent meals high in protein, and for convenience, nothing beats putting a scoop of powder in the blender with some water and pressing a button. Don't use milk for this purpose because it contains lactose, a sugar.

Yeah, your father's protein shake tasted like chalk dust, but many of today's products taste great. That's what you want, something you'll *want* to drink instead of a brew or soda.

Using supplements to lessen insulin resistance works optimally at the stage when I was taking them: early in the disease progression, before far more powerful agents—prescription drugs—are needed. And to *supplement* is precisely their role. In my mind, if exercise and diet do 90 to 95 percent of the work in defeating diabetes, supplements can add that final exclamation point. But you can pop 20 supplement pills a day, and without proper nutrition and exercise, only your wallet will become lighter.

A number of supplements seem to improve insulin sensitivity directly, while others support general health, help fuel training sessions, and so on. All of which indirectly help fight insulin resistance. Why bother with supplements when many foods contain those same nutrients? Because food isn't what it used to be. Don't get me wrong—the ideal sources of the nutrients needed to live a healthy life are whole foods, not a capsule or powder. Unfortunately, as our calories have piled up in the United States, our nourishment has dwindled. Every decade since the 1930s, the USDA has analyzed our produce in a lab, with each study finding a decline in nutritional value. Iceberg lettuce, for example, no longer contains more than trace amounts of vitamin A and folic acid, nutrients characteristic of a green leafy vegetable. They're just gone, seemingly without explanation, although some experts suggest

that farming techniques designed for quick, high-yield harvests shoulder some of the blame. Excluding the fiber, iceberg lettuce has the same
nutritional value as a piece of cardboard: zero. Since 1975, cauliflower
has lost 40 percent of its vitamin C, and broccoli, half of its calcium. In
the growing absence of these nutrients, supplements and exercise hold
ever-greater importance.

Some supplements amount to common sense. For example, nutritionists gush about a nearly miraculous enzyme found in pineapples called
bromelain, how it's so good for healing that it should be eaten in the days
before surgery. As it turns out, most of that enzyme isn't found in the
edible part but rather in the stem, the throwaway stuff. So bromelain
supplements extract those enzymes from the stem. That's logical.

A former colleague of mine at *Muscle & Fitness* named Chris Lockwood, who had become a doctoral student in exercise physiology at the
University of Oklahoma, recommended that I begin taking 7 grams of
leucine a day. Along with helping the body burn body fat, this amino
acid provokes the secretion of insulin, helping to drive more glucose and
amino acids into muscle during or after a workout, when insulin works
wonders rather than wreaking havoc. Leucine also stimulates the synthesis of the receptors responsible for channeling glucose into cells, but
you can help it out by exercising.

I began taking other supplements, including:

• Chromium (800 to 1,000 mcg daily in divided dosages, with each
meal) improves insulin sensitivity.

• The antioxidant alpha lipoic acid (600 mg per day) seems to lower
blood glucose while helping with the conversion of what you eat into
energy. Both attributes would help those with impaired glucose metabolism. Available over the counter in the United States, this blood sugar
nutrient is prescribed for diabetes, particularly neuropathy, in Europe.

• Biotin (8 to 16 grams daily) further decreases insulin resistance.

• Magnesium, according to researchers at Tufts University, improves
insulin sensitivity, which would help type 2 diabetics. Also, a study of
more than seven thousand men participating in the Honolulu Heart
Program found that a high daily intake of magnesium lessened their

chances of dying from a heart attack over fifteen- and thirty-year intervals. So I started popping 500 mg a day, in addition to the 100 mg in my multivitamin/mineral.

Bear in mind, these amounts well exceed Dietary Reference Intakes, which are based upon avoiding nutritional deficiencies. Below that threshold, specific nutritional deficiency diseases begin appearing. But the DRIs are a far cry from the *optimal* amounts for achieving maximum health in the modern world, especially as processing strips out many nutrients from whole foods.

"Fortunately, there's no way you can 'overdose' on these nutrients," says Jonny Bowden. "A doctor friend of mine regularly gives 15 grams— not micrograms—of biotin a day to blood sugar–challenged patients. Chromium, you can barely absorb anyway, and anything under 1,000 micrograms is going to be fine. And magnesium? You'd have to take grams and grams of the stuff before eliciting a negative reaction, which would be some diarrhea, worst case. Trust me, no worries on the vitamins."

Many whole, unprocessed foods such as produce and lean animal protein are great for diabetics. So are smartly engineered foods and certain dietary supplements. My diet combines all of the above. It's all the processed junk that they flank, representing the majority of the Western diet, that's turning so many Americans into type 2 diabetics.

BECAUSE THOSE UNHEALTHY foods are everywhere you look, turning your diet 180 degrees takes a concerted effort. This comes as no shock, but food packaging is designed to entice you to buy things, not to keep you healthy. When diabetics become conscious of their carb consumption for the first time, they come face-to-face with a concept called *net carbs*. I did, and it confused me. I'd reach for a product on the shelf at a convenience store that sure looked like a candy bar, only the phrase "low-carb" would be emblazoned on the package, along with a boast that it contained only 3 or 4 of these net carbs. Yet on the back I might see a listing for 17 grams of something called sugar alcohols, two words whose juxtaposition didn't strike me as the healthiest of dietary concepts. So could I tear off the wrapper and eat this thing with a clear conscience or not?

This is a fairly recent dietary dilemma. Back in simpler times, a carb was a carb. To figure out just how many of them were in a given food, chemists would do an experiment. Carbs couldn't be measured directly, but fat alone would dissolve in certain solvents, allowing a food's fat content to be measured. Protein could be measured using nitrogen: Heat the food in an oven, and the amount that evaporated could be quantified as moisture. Just like a log in a fireplace, a food's ash content— calcium, iron, and other minerals—could be determined by burning it. Carbs were simply what was left behind after everything else had been accounted for. To this day, a carbohydrate, as defined by the U.S. FDA, is that which remains in food once the fat, protein, water, and ash have been subtracted.

For much of the twentieth century, that hierarchy encompassed everything in the American diet. More recent ingredients, however, have outpaced those original rules for measuring and labeling them. This is particularly true of carbs that have been chemically modified. Consider the unique nature of glycerin, a substance hatched by food chemists, not grown by farmers. It can be analyzed like a carb in a laboratory only it doesn't behave like one inside the body. Had it existed in the early twentieth century, it, too, would have been "part of what remained."

With advances in food R&D, a carb wasn't necessarily a carb anymore. So certain makers of low-carb foods set out to recalibrate carb counts on food labels to better reflect real-world blood sugar effects. After all, that's why a guy like me pulls a low-carb product off the shelf in the first place. I don't buy an Atkins Advantage bar because it tastes better than a Butterfinger.

The net result of all this subtraction was "net carbs," a concept first used by Drs. Michael and Mary Eades in their 1996 best seller *Protein Power*. Translation: "If you're overweight or diabetic, here is the number of carbs in this product that you need to worry about." Net carbs is a marketing term rather than a legal one. The FDA requires manufacturers to list total carbs (with subtotals broken out for dietary fiber and sugars) on a product's Nutrition Facts panel. That fiber, the least carb-y carb of them all, was the first thing these companies wanted to ax. It's hard to argue with that, since fiber has no effect on blood sugar.

With rare exceptions—like the Scandinavian Bran Crispbread crackers I found on the Internet, and have shipped to me from Norway—not all sugars and other carbs can be replaced with fiber, at least not if the product is to be edible. So food scientists began to "Frankenstein" molecular structures, in order to create substances that don't raise blood sugar or hotwire insulin, yet still retain some of the sweetness and texture of good old-fashioned carbs. These were christened "low-impact carbs" and given names such as the aforementioned glycerin, polydextrose, sugar alcohols, resistant starch (a current favorite among food makers), and inulin. They allow low-carb companies to arrive at even lower net carb figures for their packaging.

Sugar alcohols don't actually contain alcohol. They're chemically modified sugars that come in nearly a dozen molecular shapes and sizes. They're still sweet, but they're converted into glucose more slowly than sugar, lowering their glycemic index and caloric content alike. The names of sugar alcohols are commonplace on the ingredients panel not only of foods but also of sugar-free gum, mouthwash, and other items.

Making these ingredients work in the real world is an experiment. Whether it's a sweet granola bar, a drink, or, say, pancakes, the ingredients must mix—both taste- and texture-wise—in a way that doesn't make someone gag. Digestion also matters. Some sugar alcohols are barely absorbed, speeding through the body . . . and right back out. Eating a chocolate bar containing 10 or 15 grams of lactitol, which is about 40 percent as sweet as sugar, might have this effect. Xylitol is barely absorbed as well, but that's used mostly in chewing gum. An amount that small doesn't upset the gastrointestinal tract.

Controversy surrounds the exclusion of sugar alcohols and similar carbs from net-carb counts. Some of these substances do raise blood glucose to varying degrees, in which case "lower-impact carbs" is more accurate than "low-impact carbs." In fact, only two sugar alcohols, erythritol and mannitol, sport a GI of zero—whereas maltitol provides enough glucose to exceed 50. Other critics of the net-carbs concept argue that a carb is indeed a carb. Many vegetables, nuts, and seeds don't jack up blood sugar, either, they note, yet those carbs are never subtracted from a carb count. "If a carb is metabolized, it needs to be counted, period, " wrote one critic.

TRUST ME. WHEN rice and hamburger buns are banned from your diet, net carbs take on their own appeal. During a trip to Wal-Mart after learning of my date with a diabetic destiny, I turned into an aisle and came upon an Atkins product line called Endulge, presumbly a contraction of *enjoy* and *indulge*. This line features low-carb doppelgängers of American snack foods, with faux sugars standing in for the real thing.

On the shelf before me were stacked boxes of Chocolate Coconut Bars, Peanut Caramel Cluster Bars, and, perhaps most audaciously, Peanut Butter Cups. If this product turned out to be truly blood sugar benign, I found myself thinking, the engineering feat would rival space flight. It's based on Hershey's Reese's Peanut Butter Cups, one of my go-to treats as a youth. When you're fourteen, the last thing you do is review the nutritional data after pulling something from a vending machine. But the adult me knows that one pack of these treats contains 260 calories, including 15 grams of fat, 180 milligrams of sodium, and 29 grams of carbs, 25 of them sugars.

But the Atkins facsimile promised not to turn my blood sugar into a Fourth of July fireworks display. According to the Nutrition Facts panel, these cups contained 18 grams of total carbs, including 4 grams of dietary fiber, 12 grams of sugar alcohols, and nary a granule of actual sugar. The net carb count was 2 grams. I was still learning the basics of carb-controlled living, but I was pretty sure that amount wouldn't kill me anytime soon.

I folded over the back of the wrapper to read the ingredients, always listed in descending order of the amount found in the product. The first entry was maltitol, a sugar alcohol. Listed fourth was the aforementioned polydextrose, another carb that wouldn't provoke my pancreas to secrete insulin.

So I took a bite. The two peanut butter cups inside didn't taste as off-putting as I thought they would. They're less sweet, to be sure, but otherwise a pretty nice stand-in for the real thing. A half an hour after eating them, my blood sugar registered 102 mg/dL. For comparison purposes, I ate the real, full-sugar version—the kind I must have eaten dozens, if not hundreds, of times over the years—at the same time, under the same circumstances, the next day. A half an hour later? My blood sugar was 132 mg/dL.

Still, the solution to America's diabetes epidemic, and to your and my health problem, doesn't lie in figuring out ways to mimic peanut butter cups and other snack foods through chemistry experiments on carbs. It sort of reminds me of the pharmaceutical approach to treating diabetes: *Eat what you want, and our pill will take care of it for you.* Here, a food scientist is playing the miracle worker.

11

LOSING THE RACE TO THE CURE

The irony is inescapable: The ADA's biggest annual fund-raising effort is a nationwide walk, called Step Out, to raise money for research into a disease that can be prevented, even reversed, by vigorous physical exercise, an antidote that historically has been given short shrift by the organization hosting the walk. If the ADA and other diabetes groups championed exercise above other diabetes therapies in the first place, donors could keep their hard-earned money, walkers could walk simply for its own sake, and we'd be doing a far, far better job of controlling type 2 diabetes than we are now.

When I first visited the home page of the ADA's Web site, I saw a photo of a heavyset African American woman slumped across the rails of a treadmill. She was drenched in sweat, looking exhausted and defeated, if not on the verge of cardiac arrest. DIET AND EXERCISE ARE NEVER EASY, read the banner headline above. EXERCISE . . . UGH! it might as well have said. I couldn't imagine a less-inviting introduction being sent to diabetics regarding the best way to save their lives and limbs.

I found a link titled FITNESS, which led me to general fitness advice and recommendations. According to the ADA, exercise is any activity that requires sufficient effort to raise heart rate and break a light sweat. You don't need a gym membership, a sports team, or fancy equipment to be physically active, they say; activities such as walking, gardening, and housework could also do the trick. They suggest doing a minimum of thirty minutes of what they define as exercise on most days, totaling about two and a half hours a week—a little more if you stretch before and after training, as they recommend. This mirrors the public-health recommendation for physical activity for everyone in the United States. In other words, as with diet, the ADA sees nothing unique about treating diabetics, that they should simply do what everyone else should do. The Web site does go on to define a comprehensive fitness routine as including aerobics, strength training, and flexibility exercises. It also suggests ways to overcome barriers to exercising, such as time limitations and fatigue.

The ADA offers all the usual caveats that accompany most exercise prescriptions: Talk to your doctor—who probably knows next to nothing about the latest in exercise science—first; start slowly; and keep water and snacks handy. Only near the end does the ADA offer a few additional tips—learn how your blood sugar responds to working out; wear a medical identification tag in case of an incident—that seem targeted to their constituency.

Diabetics never stick with their exercise regimen, goes the mantra. This argument reminds me of Dr. Westman's observations regarding doctors who blame patients for lifestyle shortcomings while failing to question their own recommendations, many of which are out of date, or plain wrong. Consider a type of exercise called high-intensity interval training, known in the field as HIIT, in which you alternate bursts of intense cardio exercise, like sprinting, with a more relaxed pace. A growing stack of studies suggests that this generates not only major cardiovascular benefits but also better glycemic improvements than steady-state cardio does (e.g., running at the same pace). Furthermore, it takes a fraction of the two and a half hours a week of workout time recommended for diabetics in guidelines such as the ADA's. Only no one with a real platform is telling this to type 2 diabetics.

HIIT prompts striking physiological adaptations. Recently, a research team from Heriot-Watt University in Edinburgh, Scotland, launched a study with men in their twenties who were sedentary but outwardly healthy. Even before the experiment started, however, their metabolic response to a carb-loaded drink showed blood sugar problems brewing. The young men were already becoming insulin resistant. They just didn't know it yet.

In the experiment, some male subjects did HIIT training and others did conventional aerobic training. The HIIT-training group alternated thirty seconds of fast pedaling on an exercise bike with four minutes of rest, which is a pretty modest ratio. They completed four of those thirty-second sets each workout, and three such workouts per week.

After only two weeks, the spike in their blood glucose after the sugary drink had diminished more in the HIIT group than in the traditional cardio group. Better yet, it took 23 percent less insulin production by the pancreas to lower their blood sugar, a signal that their insulin resistance was improving more in less exercise time than their counterparts. Not a bad payoff for a total of six minutes of exercise a week.

I asked James Timmons, Ph.D., a professor in the university's school of engineering and physical sciences, and the experiment's lead investigator, for an explanation regarding results that sound counterintuitive: less work, better results. "The intense contractions that fatigue muscles really break down carbohydrate stores in muscle as well," he says. "The muscles then become much more responsive to insulin as they attempt to replenish these stores."

Unfortunately, the prevailing diabetes guidelines focus on moderate aerobic training, such as walking and, er, housecleaning. Sure, cleaning may have been aerobic for your great-grandmother when she was washing the floor on her hands and knees, but vacuum cleaners, dishwashers, and other labor-saving devices have taken the elbow grease out of housework, along with much of its benefit as physical activity. You're going to need to do more than push a broom to sweep away diabetes.

"[More casual training] may be good for some cardiovascular endpoints, but we do not believe that it is optimal, either in terms of time or the metabolic effect achieved," says Timmons. Other recent studies, including one published in the official journal of the American Heart Association, found that when it comes to fighting diabetes, more intense training trumps more casual training.

"Clearly, diabetes is one of the biggest risk factors for cardiovascular disease," says Timmons. "This is what diabetics usually die of. So the best exercise protocol to optimally combat insulin resistance is an important thing to identify. We think that the United States and United Kingdom guidelines are out of date and do not reflect decades of known physiology." No one's recommending that a diabetic grandmother on insulin and six other meds, as well as extensive complications, hit the treadmill like an Olympic sprinter. But with a doctor's okay, the protocol can be modified, allowing even those who are quite ill to intensify their training over time relative to their baseline. For the rest of the more than eighty million diabetics and prediabetics across the country, shouldn't someone be telling them that, if nothing else, they can improve their insulin sensitivity and glucose metabolism by exercising vigorously for *4 percent* of the time recommended in the current guidelines? Isn't that preferable to assuming that diabetics will fail to invest two and a half hours in training, and prescribing a bunch of meds in anticipation of that failure?

"The more you do, the better off you are," says the University of South Carolina's Blair of diabetics and exercise. Any effort should be encouraged, any success applauded. But the point is that diabetics may not have to work out as long as they think they do in order to tap into exercise's magical metabolic benefits. For many, the efficiency of HIIT would prove very appealing. It's about giving diabetics the full array of options, and letting them choose the ones that fit their lifestyle.

When patients feel like they're achieving fast results through efficient means, they're more likely to keep at it. After all, it's working for them. As a writer in the ADA's own journal *Clinical Diabetes* notes, "[I]f a behavior, such as exercising, leads to desired benefits, the behavior is reinforced and thus is more likely to be repeated. If, on the other hand, exercise fails to gain benefit or is seen as punishing, it diminishes in value and thus is not likely to be repeated."

Punishing—as in the woman slumped over the treadmill.

ALONG WITH A low-carb eating plan, a gym membership is the most potent antidote to type 2 diabetes. Experts in the diabetes field have knock-down-drag-out debates over everything imaginable—except the benefit of exercise. The research is unequivocal. For example, a major Finnish study on diabetes prevention found that regular exercise reduced diabetes incidence in subjects by nearly 70 percent compared with subjects who didn't exercise. What's more, a follow-up done three years after the active phase of the study found a 36 percent reduction in diabetes among the group that had exercised and dieted. This belies the notion about people not sticking with the program.

As Blair said during a presentation I attended, diabetics shouldn't need a note from their doctor *to* exercise, as the disclaimers usually suggest. They should need a note *not* to.

Weight loss improves glucose control and insulin sensitivity, and exercise helps with weight loss. Diabetics should be hitting their stride and lifting weights if only for that reason. But like low-carb dieting, exercise improves insulin sensitivity even without weight loss. In the Diabetes Prevention Program, those subjects who didn't hit their target for weight loss, yet did hit their target for exercise, still had a 44 percent reduction in diabetes risk relative to a placebo group.

The liver reacts to exercise by breaking down glycogen, those stored carbs. At the same time, cells become more proficient at absorbing glucose from the bloodstream, like they're supposed to. The increased uptake tends to exceed the increased production. When it does, blood sugar levels drop.

That's not all, though. As the HIIT researcher Timmons suggested, simply by contracting vigorously, muscles are primed to absorb blood glucose with or without insulin's help. "Exercise engages the glucose transporters that sit inside your cells to go to the membrane through a different signaling mechanism than insulin, but it accomplishes the same thing," says the University of Connecticut's Volek. "The neat thing is that in diabetics, this exercise-stimulating pathway remains intact and healthy even as the insulin-signaling pathway becomes more garbled."

Looking for the cure for type 2 diabetes? This is it.

While exercise revs up the body's metabolic machinery it also elevates mood, which makes dietary compliance that much easier. Not only that, but it also encourages an aggressive mind-set. Instead of letting the disease run its course, exercisers are taking preemptive action. Rather than sitting on their backside, they're kicking ass.

Working out is an essential long-term strategy for type 2 diabetics, but when a patient asks their doctor or an endocrinologist what they should actually, like, *do*, a blank stare is often the response. When prescribing a diabetes drug, a doctor won't just tell a patient to take it—and then leave it to them to come up with a dosage, decide how often to take it, and learn about interactions with other drugs and foods. The doctor, or more likely the pharmacist who fills the 'scrip, will provide clear written instructions.

But with exercise, should you be running twenty minutes once a day, or ten minutes twice a day? How about intervals—should you try those? Should you be lifting weights? What rep range? How often? What should you eat before you train? What should you eat while you train? What should you eat after you train? What about proper technique? Injury prevention is critical. If a diabetic blows out a shoulder or knee doing something incorrectly in the gym, then they can't work out; and if they can't work out, they won't remain healthy. This is life-and-death stuff we're talking about.

Diabetics, especially, need exercise recommendations specific to their medical condition. "You shouldn't just say, 'Okay, go to a gym and start training for forty-five minutes or an hour,'" says James E. Wright, Ph.D., who served as chief of the exercise science branch of the U.S. Army Physical Fitness School, and was later a colleague of mine at *Muscle & Fitness*. "It doesn't work, because people aren't used to it. The first rule in fitness is, 'Be there.' The goal of every workout must be to make the person come back for the next workout. Consistency is the key."

Unfortunately, short of hiring a personal trainer—who may know as little about diabetes as your doctor knows about exercise—you're on your own. When I was first diagnosed with prediabetes, I had the advantage of having worked at a muscle magazine for nearly a decade, and at a health magazine for four months. So I thought of ways to combine various things I had learned into what struck me as a coherent strategy. I'd torch any excess sugar that remained from my low-carb diet by working out six times a week—superset-based weight-lifting sessions (no standing around between exercises) one day, cardio intervals (those short bursts punctuated with downshifts) the next. On low carbs, presumably I wasn't storing much glycogen, the body's main fuel source, so I'd have to hit it hard and fast.

The only time I'd favor simple sugars—chocolate milk, yogurt, a piece of fruit—would be right before, during, or right after my workout. "If you're doing weights or cardio, you'll be using those carbs," my nutritionist friend Mohr had told me.

THE HIGH FREQUENCY of my workouts turned out to be dialed in perfectly. The blood sugar–impaired are far better off working out for half an hour, five or six days a week, than they are biking for, say, three hours on a Sunday. Score another point for intervals. At that training frequency, an hour a day for exercise might be hard to find.

Braun has been studying relationships among insulin resistance, diabetes, and exercise for nearly two decades. One freezing morning in January 2008, we met in his office down the hall from the energy metabolism laboratory he runs at the University of Massachusetts in Amherst. For those who can't handle sugar and other carbs, he, too, likens exercise to a prescription drug. "You can take more or less of it, but like any drug, the effect wanes, so you have to take it again," he says. The salutary effects of exercise on insulin sensitivity end twenty-four to forty-eight hours after a workout. So you want a measured dose of this medicine, exercise, hitting your system nearly every day. With a drug, you wouldn't skip six days and then pop a week's worth of pills all at once, would you?

In experiments, Braun finds it easy to wreck the insulin sensitivity of even his physically fit subjects. He need only overfeed them and turn off the treadmill, and insulin resistance reappears. But fit people who resume exercising and dieting recover as fast as they backslid. In contrast, the lower a person's fitness level, the slower their recovery. "The fit already have all the metabolic machinery to recover quickly," says Braun, referring to mitochondria and oxidative enzymes. "We just 'suspended' them for a while." The take-home: Establish a base fitness level and improve from there. Even if the effects of a single exercise bout on insulin sensitivity have a druglike half-life, you're building sweat equity against diabetes because of this long-term conditioning effect.

Correct dosing for exercise can vary by individual; humans don't respond with the consistency of mutant lab mice. For the first year or so postdiagnosis, thirty minutes a day worked great for me, and was about all I felt like I could do. Three and a half low-carb years later, I like to hit it hard for forty minutes a day, six days a week. That's because at the forty-five-minute mark, I'm ready to drop. My low-carb diet allows for only so much glycogen storage. When it's gone, I'm done. You may need fifteen minutes a day, or twenty, or forty. Your body will tell you. Make sure you're listening.

When I told Braun about my initial self-styled approach of alternating three days of weight supersets with three days of cardio intervals, he liked the idea. "That makes perfect sense to me," he said. "It stresses different metabolic pathways. That should work for 95 percent of those individuals with blood sugar issues." It sure worked for me.

Based on interviews I had done with exercise physiologists as part of my job, I already knew how effective and efficient interval training was at boosting cardiovascular fitness. When I interviewed Braun, I asked whether intervals might also have positive effects on glucose control, of the sort that Timmons and his group had found in Scotland. "There's a certain logic to expending energy at a higher rate for a shorter period of time, in terms of elevated heart rate and positive adaptations from the stress on muscles and bones," Braun had said. "What you've been doing is trading duration for intensity. The research is showing that you can do that and achieve similar benefits."

What Braun meant about the duration-for-intensity trade is that for improving insulin sensitivity and glucose metabolism, total calorie expenditure is what matters—not how you expend those calories. So let's say you and I are both diabetics, and we want to help our blood sugar by burning 200 calories after dinner. I decide to hop on the treadmill and go like a bat out of hell for ten minutes. You decide to go for an hour-and-a-half stroll with your wife or husband. Well, if we both burn 200 calories, we've achieved the same positive blood sugar effect. That's been the prevailing theory in recent years.

That alone would be great news, especially during a time crunch. You can be as efficient as you want, really. But as it turns out, the latest studies suggest that the blood sugar benefits of high-intensity training don't just meet those of longer, steady-pace cardio sessions—they exceed them. Apparently even when the calories burned are equal, training more intensely offers diabetics a bonus.

This hearkens back to what Timmons and his group found. "The use of muscle glycogen is very intensity dependent," says Sheri Colberg-Ochs, Ph.D., professor of exercise science at Old Dominion University, and a type 1 diabetic. "The higher the intensity, the faster the rate at which you use it." The less glycogen stored in muscles, the more receptive those muscles seem to be to taking sugar from the blood for glycogen storage.

Exercising with greater intensity isn't limited to sprinting full bore on a treadmill, although that's great if you can do it. It could mean taking a section of your evening walk—say, the distance between two mailboxes on a country road, or between light poles in the city or suburbs—and stepping up your pace for that interval. Colberg-Ochs finds that once diabetics start with even small intensity bumps like that, they often pick up their pace more overall. Training more intensely becomes contagious. Again, because it produces results.

ANOTHER CONSIDERATION IS the ideal workout time for maintaining stable blood sugar. This hasn't been studied much, but I asked Braun for an educated guess. "I think it's partly a matter of preference, but exercising in the morning gives you all day to bring your physical activity and calories into some sort of balance," he says. "If you exercise at night and then follow that with a meal, you don't have the same opportunity to expend that energy [you've consumed]."

He continues: "There's so little data, but I think we all have this suspicion that eating a bunch of calories and then going to bed can't possibly be good. It seems like that would be the optimal condition for fat storage." That was a wake-up call for me, since I'd always trained up until my gym's closing time.

If the central preoccupation of exercise for diabetics is how many calories a workout burns, how much of that energy should they put back inside their body? At *Muscle & Fitness*, we preached taking in simple sugars as soon as the last set or sprint ended, when the body wants to store carbs in muscle as glycogen. Bodybuilders *wanted* an insulin surge driving nutrients into those training-primed muscles.

But what should I do now? Since I was insulin resistant, wouldn't those carbs be rebuffed by my cells and remain stranded in my blood, where I didn't want them? Or should I take advantage of increased insulin sensitivity postexercise and try to jam glycogen into cells while I could? That way, I'd have energy reserves to draw upon during my next workout. Or would filling up those stores only make it harder for me to handle sugar at other times during the day?

I had a lot of questions. Answers were in shorter supply. Erring on the low-carb side, I opted for a protein shake containing single-digit carb amounts, or none at all. That protein would at least help my muscle tissue recover from the training session, without provoking an excessive insulin response. That was my rationale anyway.

Near the end of our visit, I mentioned this quandary to Braun. I probably shouldn't have been surprised that he had not only thought about the dilemma before but also studied it. Going into the experiment he designed, he expected to find that not only *what* you eat but also *when* you eat it relative to a workout would dictate glucose tolerance and insulin sensitivity. "We thought that eating immediately postexercise would be very different than waiting three hours," says Braun. "That if you ate immediately postexercise, you'd store lots of glycogen, like athletes do on purpose, and that would really impair your insulin sensitivity. We thought that for people who were insulin resistant, the recommendation would be reversed: *Don't* eat right after you exercise."

That wasn't the case, however. As it turned out, the timing of that consumption makes only a subtle difference. What was critically important, though, was the total amount of carbs in that postworkout meal. When the just-expended energy was "fed back" after a workout, the insulin resistant whose calories came from protein and fat were more insulin sensitive than those who consumed carbs—even when total calories were the same. So my postworkout protein shake is just what the doctor should have ordered. The same dichotomy applies between the trained and untrained, by the way. The better shape you're in, the more carbs your body can absorb postworkout without insulin sensitivity suffering.

"As long as you don't replenish your glycogen levels after exercise, the improvement in insulin sensitivity lingers," says Volek. "It's yet another reason why low-carb diets work so well for diabetics." What's the payoff? Burn 500 calories on the treadmill without replacing them, and your insulin sensitivity jumps 40 percent! More insulin sensitivity means less insulin output. The pancreas senses the job is being completed and eventually stops. Remember, too much insulin can damage arteries and perhaps stimulate cancer cell growth. The more insulin sensitive that tissues are, the better.

I WAS MAKING a big mistake in training late, slugging down a drink containing several dozen grams of fast-acting sugars, and then falling asleep. Based on what I had read about sports nutrition—not to mention all those commercials I had seen showing Gatorade-drenched athletes training like future Olympic gold medalists—I thought I needed that stuff. But I was struck by how little effect *not* drinking that sugar water had on my more recent workouts, the ones performed on a low-carb diet. Of all the self-experimentation I've done since being diagnosed as prediabetic, this realization surprised me the most.

I asked Braun why shifting my fuel mix had seemed so easy. He believes that while you can't replace carbs entirely with fat, you can shift your metabolism. "I think [consuming carbs during a workout is] not the end-all of athletic performance, as some of the major purveyors of carbohydrate-containing compounds [Gatorade and others] and most of the popular press would have you believe," he says. "There's been this idea that if you don't drink carbohydrates during exercise, you won't be able to finish your workout. So now people won't go anywhere or do anything without a sports drink or an energy bar. Do you need all that stuff? The answer is almost certainly no. Some of these products have so many carbs that if you consume [them] after working out, you actually end up with a net gain of energy." For a diabetic, especially, that defeats the purpose of the workout.

If you train, your heart will thank you for the effort because revving it up once a day in the gym allows it to work less hard during the remaining twenty-three and a half hours. As it turns out, diabetics who exercise tend to have lower heart rates and blood pressure (both at rest and while exercising) and increased stroke volume and cardiac output than diabetics who remain sedentary—sitting ducks for diabetes.

Sometimes we forget that our heart isn't made of glass, that it's actually a muscle. Conceivably, exercise might improve the insulin sensitivity of this life-giving muscle itself. But exercise's bigger impact on cardiovascular health comes from its effects on the energy metabolism of the larger skeletal muscles: the pectorals (chest), quadriceps (thighs), and so on. Collectively, they have the capacity to keep excess glucose out of the bloodstream, taking pressure off the heart. If your heart also becomes more insulin sensitive, consider it a bonus.

One way diabetes damages the heart is through a condition called left ventricular diastolic dysfunction (LVDD). "It's the most common feature of the diabetic heart," Johns Hopkins's Stewart told his audience at the ADA conference I attended in New Orleans. "It markedly increases the risk of heart failure."

I'm simplifying here, but in LVDD, the left ventricle doesn't refill with blood properly after each pump of the heart. This refilling process can be measured by something called the E:A ratio, which has to do with the amount of blood-filling that occurs early versus late in the heart-pumping cycle. In a healthy heart, this ratio is above 1, not below it.

A study led by Stewart sought to measure the effect of exercise on this ratio. The participants were diabetics, average age fifty-seven, who were relatively free from complications: no insulin required as of yet, no history or clinical symptoms of cardiovascular disease. They were obese, though, and their average E:A ratio was .95, a level that represents modest LVDD. Clearly their hearts were not in anything approaching perfect working order.

Over six months, some of the diabetics followed a supervised exercise program of cardio and weights. *Very* moderate work—we're not talking Tour de France or Mr. Olympia prep here. Like clockwork, the usual sorts of benefits appeared: less body fat, increased strength, improved lung capacity. What's more, their E:A ratios rose to 1.05, on average, as their dysfunctional hearts began to heal. In contrast, the E:A ratio of a sedentary control group deteriorated to .91.

As Stewart outlined during his presentation, three other diabetic-heart killers include damage to the inner lining of arteries; a stiffening of those arteries; and chronic, systemic inflammation. Studies that he highlighted in his talk suggest that exercise is a formidable defense against all three of these threats. The cells that line the arteries seem to be a key intersection between diabetes and heart disease. These cells compose a thin layer, called endothelium, which isn't just a coating for arterial walls; it also helps regulate blood pressure and limit inflammation by releasing a chemical called nitric oxide. HDL is deemed "good" cholesterol in part because it stimulates nitric oxide release, although this ability seems to diminish in diabetics. The need to keep HDL working on your behalf is yet another reason why prevention is so important.

High blood sugar and excessive insulin can damage endothelial cells, causing them to malfunction. When that happens, nitric oxide production decreases. Cardiovascular disease helps fill the void.

Exercising actually triggers the endothelial cells to release nitric oxide, allowing blood passageways to expand as needed. That's much better than those passageways becoming constricted or even closing off. When vessels expand, blood flows unimpeded. So in essence, every workout for your lungs is a workout for your arteries, too.

A University of Maryland study found that when a group of diabetics (average age, fifty-two years) followed an exercise program for eight weeks, an ultrasound-based measurement of flow-mediated dilation—an excellent indicator of endothelial function—increased by a whopping 200 percent!

FOR DECADES, SO-CALLED diabetes experts cringed at the thought of diabetics picking up a barbell. As did many cardiologists. Not only did the experts think that lifting weights wouldn't help, but they also thought it might put diabetics at risk for some sort of vascular event. You know, the Big One, boom, right there under the barbell. But this is one prescription that actually works.

"Swallowing a pill is easier," says David J. Dyck, Ph.D., associate professor in human health and nutritional sciences at the University of Guelph, and a top researcher in the field of exercise and insulin resistance. "But as long as that attitude pervades our society, we're in a lot of trouble. It's amazing how something as simple and modest as a bit of exercise can do so much with so few side effects."

If the calories burned are the same, resistance training equals aerobic exercise at improving insulin resistance and glucose control. In fact, weight training offers a bonus to the glucose-impaired: It burns fat and builds muscle. Remember, muscle is a storage depot for glycogen, those carbs that are packed away. Exercise creates more muscle tissue and insulin receptors, improving the absorption of glucose into muscles. They suck it up like a sponge. And muscle tissue is where glucose should be, not floating in your blood or being converted into fat for lack of glycogen storage space. The loss of muscle that comes with aging may go a long way toward explaining why insulin resistance seems to worsen over time.

As muscle absorbs all that glucose, the pancreas can breathe a giant sigh of relief. "For a given glucose load, the pancreas doesn't pump out as much insulin in a trained person as it does for an untrained person," says Wright.

In 1997, the American College of Sports Medicine (ACSM) and ADA released a joint position paper on diabetes and exercise that didn't mention resistance training. In 2000, ACSM released a new position stand without the ADA, mentioning resistance training but not emphasizing it. For its part, the ADA revised its exercise recommendations to include resistance training along with aerobic exercise only in 2006. That was many years after the benefits were obvious, especially to anyone who happened to lift weights after developing blood sugar problems. "Things move slowly in the world of academic medicine," says Braun, putting it kindly. As Blair points out, this past decade has witnessed an explosion in exercise-related research. There's now a nice-size chunk regarding the effects of exercise on insulin resistance and type 2 diabetes. The ADA's official guidelines on exercise and diabetes, which were perfunctory to begin with, incorporate little of this new research.

Type 2 diabetes is a lifestyle disease, one that can be prevented and maybe even reversed by exercising. Exercise science should be the centerpiece of our diabetes guidance, not a few paragraphs of boilerplate that change imperceptibly from one year to the next and lag the latest research by a decade. If one goal for diabetics is to burn as many calories lifting weights as they do when performing aerobic exercises, then why is there no discussion of circuit training or supersets, both of which were invented ages ago to elevate heart rate and burn calories? Those two resistance-training styles are perfect for type 2 diabetics. Will they receive a line or two of ink in the guidelines of 2020?

If diabetes threatens your health, don't wait another decade for the diabetes authorities to reach a consensus about intervals or circuit training. Exercise science isn't rocket science. Diabetics should exercise frequently, consistently, and intensely, but not endlessly. Get in, hit it hard, and get out. Avoid skipping even two days in a row. Treat exercise like you would a prescription drug; your life is at stake. Only this prescription works, and the side effects—weight loss, mood elevation, and so on—are all positive.

AFTER A DAY filled with ten hours of work, dietary diligence, and a hard workout, I might have thought my skirmish with diabetes would be over by 11:00 P.M., at least until the next morning. Instead, another phase was just beginning. Actually, of all the lifestyle adjustments I had to make, sleep was the one where I fell short the most.

Any large house built in 1912—after its predecessor burned down—has a voice all its own. That's true of where I lived, especially during a Pennsylvania winter, when snowdrifts soundproof the mill from the outside world. Inside, beams settle. Heat pipes groan. According to local legend, ghosts haunt the four stories of the mill, which was converted into a single-family residence in the 1950s. There was the young woman whose body was dumped by the railroad tracks next to the property in what was the Lehigh Valley's version of L.A.'s Black Dahlia murder. Then there was Wolfgang Schlegel, the eccentric engineer who managed to rebuild the stone dam while owning the mill back in the 1980s. That is, before he plunged to his death while chipping ice off the waterwheel behind the house.

Never a sound sleeper, I would wake up three or four times a night at the mill. Sometimes a creak or clank would startle me, but at other times the awakenings seemed spontaneous. In reality, my own hypoglycemic body was craving sugar, even from deepest sleep. As blood sugar drops during the night, the brain detects the change and dials its own 911. It's a classic diabetes dilemma: You need sleep, but hypoglycemia wakes you up in the middle of the night, interrupting this essential health tonic. This disease is nothing if not clever.

Poor sleep is a nightmare for your glucose metabolism, helping to sow the seeds for diabetes. Even one night of partial sleep reduces insulin sensitivity in a healthy person, so you can imagine what chronic tossing and turning does to someone whose glucose tolerance is already impaired. "Diabetes and chronic loss of sleep share the fact that both affect millions and one is detrimental to the other," according to Brazilian researchers. "Indeed, sleep deficits . . . foster metabolic syndrome that culminates in sleep disorders like Restless Legs Syndrome and sleep apnea, which in turn lead to poor sleep quality."

The relationship between sleep apnea—breathing interruptions that occur during sleep—and diabetes is particularly incestuous. Sleep apnea increases the risk of metabolic syndrome and diabetes, but these two conditions are often associated with obesity, which in turn raises the risk of sleep apnea. Talk about a vicious circle.

AS WINTER GAVE way to the first signs of spring, any sluggishness in response to training while on low carbs vanished. I felt like my body was undergoing a reawakening of its own. All the things I was doing to ward off diabetes weren't a drag; they were rocket boosters. I *loved* this new lifestyle. If I was on a date, like I was one spring evening, the influence of diabetes on my life amounted to ordering my burger without the bun and replacing fries with a Caesar salad without the croutons. That's not my idea of personal sacrifice. Every meal doesn't have to produce a gastric orgasm when you're eating as frequently as I do and living the rest of your life to the fullest.

By thinking otherwise, our nation confers so much power upon type 2 diabetes that it's unworthy of wielding. We're indoctrinated to think that it always wins in the end, when it should lose every single time. Our collective response to this lifestyle disease is to fill drug prescriptions? Shouldn't the land of the free and the home of the brave set its sights much higher than that? We defeated the Third Reich, but we can't beat *this*?

Beating back diabetes isn't about deprivation; it's about enrichment. In truth, you're asked to give up nothing that matters in life. Not even the bottle of cabernet I was sharing on my second date with Natasha. As our glasses clinked, it dawned on me how effortless and organic beating this disease can become once your lifestyle makes sense for your body—how it can't even enter unless you lay out a welcome mat. You want to avoid beers that aren't "light" and sugary elixirs, like those

Bourbon Street daiquiris, but wine, drunk in moderation, may actually be good for the glucose intolerant. It certainly doesn't seem to harm blood sugar.

If I'm on a date, I don't want to be ordering a Diet Coke with dinner. And when you're winning this fight, even moderation can take the occasional night off.

Our dinner was served on a balcony in Jim Thorpe, a small Alpine-like village near the Pocono Mountains that draws Pennsylvania bikers rather than skiers. Afterward, Natasha asked me if I wanted to go to a lake outside of town that she remembered from high school. We drove through warm spring darkness until a sign appeared. She recognized it and told me to turn off. We wound our way back to a deserted parking lot. After we exited the car, she led me back through a thicket of tall trees. It was midnight now, and we had arrived at the edge of a deserted lake. It would have been pitch-black out without the moon's beam and a blanket of stars illuminating our surroundings.

At that moment, my prediabetic universe consisted only of darkness, the heavens, the distant *whoosh* of a waterfall, the sound of a million frogs croaking in unison, and this gorgeous young woman standing at the water's edge like a forest nymph.

"Have you ever gone skinny-dipping before?" she asked me over her shoulder.

I thought for a split second. Aside from my morning shower, I don't think I had been fully naked in water for a decade or more. By the time I told her that, um, no, I hadn't, she'd stripped bare and was wading waist deep into the lake, keeping her back to me and placing her forearms across her chest whenever she turned to speak over her shoulder. Her laughter would erupt like a volcano, shoot up into the night sky, and explode there like a fireworks display.

"C'mon," she said, laughing even harder. After a brief silence, she began singing a torch song to the frogs in the hills around us.

I ditched my clothes on the shore and waded in, too, although Natasha had drifted farther away from me. Feeling the cold water against my skin and mud oozing around my feet and ankles as they sank, hearing her serenade, I realized how divorced I had been from the natural

world for much of my adult life. Before I discovered that my very survival hung in the balance, I'd had little connection with what I ate or
where it came from, or with the kind of physical conditioning that
would have been required back when humans needed to use their body
to hunt or forage for food, rather than feeding coins into a vending machine or phoning Domino's.

"I want you to just scream," she yelled over.

"What are you talking about?" I asked, chest-deep in the lake now,
feeling my arms pulling through the water in what felt like slow motion, the two glasses of cab still humming through my body.

"Haven't you ever just screamed at the top of your lungs?"

Natasha turned back away from me, and, moments later, let out a
primal roar that seemed destined for the moon and stars. Maybe it
reached that far, although I suspect only the frogs and I heard it.

My turn had come. I took a deep breath, summoned every ounce of
energy I could from my diaphragm and lungs, and let out a yell that
made it only across the lake before falling back to earth.

But it was a start.

12

A SINKING FEELING

By the spring of 2007, I felt as if I was overriding my own genetic predisposition, the same one that, left unaccounted for, had been my father's undoing. Denying a disease can be easier than confronting it, and he chose the former. So do many people, and not just of his generation. I suspect that my father's mind-set was similar to that of a twenty-something friend of mine who often ignores a serious heart condition. "People die in hospitals," she says, and it's a hard point to counter. Plus my father had obviously led a busy life, fathering seven children and starting and running several businesses. His health was never his highest priority, I'm guessing.

In light of my prediabetes diagnosis, I felt like I had to make it mine. Presented with a harbinger of what doctors tell us is an incurable disease, I had defied conventional wisdom and jerry-rigged my own action plan, integrating cutting-edge information from the realms of nutrition, exercise science, sleep research, and other disciplines. I certainly *felt* better, but could some of that be a placebo effect? Or would the same tests that had indicated prediabetes now confirm that these strategies were producing real results?

I scheduled my first blood draw since September 2006, when I was diagnosed. A reading below 100 on the fasting plasma glucose test had been a Holy Grail of sorts for me from the beginning of this odyssey. As the day of my appointment neared, I hawk-eyed my carb counts more than usual. I put extra oomph into my workouts, adding extra intervals to each session and banging out more reps at the end of weight sessions. When the day arrived, I left work and headed over to Dr. H.'s office.

A nurse drew my blood and sent me on my way.

A week and a half later, I found myself back at Dr. H.'s office. This time, he smiled when he opened the manila folder. Over the past six months, my fasting glucose had fallen from 116 to 102, leaving me a mere two points above the prediabetes threshold. My triglycerides had fallen from 298 to 89, well below the upper limit of 150 for healthy levels of these blood fats. My A1C was 5, a number that supposedly indicates an absence of diabetes. Perhaps most telling, my fasting insulin level stood at 2.9 microunits per milliliter (mcU/mL). This hadn't been measured back in the fall, but it was actually *below* the normal range of 5 to 20 mcU/mL. If you think of the pancreas as the spigot for insulin, mine had gone from gushing out of control to nearly off. Only small, measured amounts were being secreted. That meant *I* was now at the controls of the hormone that had been turning me diabetic.

While my fasting glucose was still on the high side, my A1C was in the desirable range. The A1C reflected my blood sugar's behavior round the clock for at least the past three months, maybe more. By this seemingly foolproof measure, my blood sugar wasn't just nondiabetic—it was nearly perfect.

After we wrapped up the review of my results, I rose to leave, and Dr. H. patted me on the back as I headed out the door. "You've proven that this problem can be addressed with diet and exercise," he said. "Most of my patients don't do that. You are to be commended."

I was relieved. Still, something didn't feel right. For all of my efforts over the preceding six months, my fasting glucose score was still high. What's more, if my A1C number was normal, and my insulin was actually low, why was my fasting number still prediabetic? Taken together, these numbers didn't seem to add up, although I didn't know enough to know why. My doctor wasn't going tell me. He didn't know, either.

For assurance, I thought back to a question I had asked Dr. Deeb during our interview. I had asked him if a normal A1C was a sure sign of blood sugar being well under control. If anyone should know, surely it was a member of the ADA's national leadership. "Yes, you would definitely be getting good blood sugars at home if you had a normal A1C."

But something was nagging at me. It was time for a third opinion.

"ACTUALLY, THIS IS really bad."

The voice on the other end of the line belonged to Dr. Berkowitz of the Center for Balanced Health in New York City, to whom I had faxed my blood work. These same scores had prompted my family physician to pat me on the back, congratulate me on a job well done, and send me on my way. Dr. Berkowitz had taken one look at them and arrived at a different conclusion.

He had only a fax of my test results. He had never examined me. He had never met me nor seen my photograph. He wasn't looking at someone tall, thin, and, from all appearances, healthy. He was looking at a sheet of paper suggesting metabolic problems as serious as those shadowing an overweight person on the verge of diabetes. Immediately he had seen what he called "a big red flag." My A1C score, the blood sugar benchmark, appeared normal, but my fasting glucose reading was still high. Mathematics told Dr. Berkowitz that for this to be the case, my blood sugar must be too low at other times.

"The problem is that the fasting score doesn't give you a lot of information," he said. "Your A1C, 5, suggests a fasting blood sugar reading of 80, but instead that's 102. So there have to be some 60s to balance out the 100s. I think your biggest problem is hypoglycemia—low blood sugar."

Dr. Berkowitz also suggested that these swings between high and low blood sugar lay at the root of my high blood pressure and high resting heart rate. "Think how much harder your body has to work because of that roller-coaster ride," he said.

To assess my metabolic health, Dr. Berkowitz invited me to come down to his office and take a glucose-tolerance test. He would do a stress test on my metabolic system by giving me a sugary drink and mapping my blood sugar response by drawing blood on the half hour. It made sense to me. After all, they diagnose heart disease with a stress test.

In May 2007 I arrived at his office in midtown Manhattan for my sugar stress test. Dr. Berkowitz treats people who, like me, have abnormal blood sugar. Everyone has some peculiar passion or obsession in life, and Dr. Berkowitz's is blood sugar curves. He speaks of the unusual ones revealed by blood tests with the mixture of awe and wonder an astronomer might use to convey the peculiarities of a constellation. "I see people who drop 150 points on a glucose-tolerance test!" he blurts, sounding geeked by the challenge this presents. "Those are the hardest cases because of the rapid change."

We talked for a bit. Then Dr. Berkowitz, a mild-mannered maverick who is balding and wears wire-framed glasses, handed me off to an assistant. She presented me with a small plastic container and then directed me to the bathroom. My urine sample would tell the doctor if sugar was "spilling"; remember, peeing is one way the body rids itself of excess glucose. Even in ancient times, healers noticed that ants would make a beeline to a diabetic's urine. I'd later be told that, indeed, I was spilling, although no doubt less than I would have been without my diet-and-exercise regimen.

The test would be administered in a nondescript room. I was going to have my blood drained periodically for the next five hours by a nurse who was pretty and pleasant. The good doctor handed me a clipboard. He wanted me to write down how I felt every half hour, intervals that would correspond to the nurse's blood draws. Unlike most physicians, who just poke their patients with needles and read the numbers, Dr. Berkowitz wants to know how his patients feel inside at a given moment during the test. I would find out why later, when we reviewed the results.

After some prep work, the nurse stuck me; this first measurement would record my fasting state. Then she served me breakfast: a glass of orange goop, 75 grams of glucose, roughly the amount contained in two cans of regular soda. I slugged it down. At first, nothing felt different, and my initial scribblings on the doctor's clipboard were about as interesting as phone book entries. I set down the clipboard and picked up a magazine. Only later would I discover that my blood sugar had already leaped well into prediabetic territory, a postmeal spike that sets the stage for heart disease. My blood sugar was high, but I felt normal. That's the kicker. If I didn't know any better, I'd go through my adult life triggering three or four spikes a day, damaging my heart until, one day, a doctor would be telling me I needed bypass surgery—if I were lucky. Otherwise I'd slump over at my desk one day, dead, or fall asleep and never wake up.

During the test's second hour, I became groggy, even though I had slept pretty well overnight. I couldn't stifle yawns. Even having the older gentleman seated nearby introduce himself as Theodore Bear ("My friends call me Teddy," he said with a smile) couldn't elicit a chuckle, so buzzed was I from the sugar drink. Then, around the two-hour mark, I became nervous and agitated; my hand felt a little shaky when I reached for the pencil tied to the clipboard.

For the remainder of the test, I didn't feel agitated, just sluggish, like I was trying to wake up all over again.

Finally, mercifully, the test came to an end. "That's enough torture for one day," said Dr. Berkowitz, his attempt at metabolic mirth. He promised to be in touch.

I stepped onto the street below, made my way around a corner, and ducked into the first restaurant I saw. I ordered a chicken breast, vegetables, and a glass of wine, even though the doc had advised against drinking alcohol after the test. I didn't care. I was famished, not having eaten since the night before; even the sugar swill was five hours ago. My blood sugar was still low, and my brain knew what it wanted—the bread the waiter had left on the table. I resisted the temptation, knowing the trap. That "eat when you're hungry" advice doled out to type 2 diabetics by many dietitians is so misguided. Once hunger arrives, your brain, in search of a quick sugar fix, will make you reach for the last thing you should have at that moment—even if it should know better because of the knowledge stored there. This is more primal.

A WEEK AFTER taking my glucose-tolerance test, I picked up the phone in my office at *Men's Health*. Dr. Berkowitz was on the line. He wanted to review my test results in person, and I didn't press him for a preview of coming attractions. Like airline pilots speaking from a cockpit, doctors on the phone communicate by tone as well as by words. My new doctor's tone didn't alarm me. Not yet anyway.

If my blood sugar was behaving normally, from start to finish, over five hours, it should have traveled within a range of 35 points, going no higher than 120 and no lower than 85. Dr. Berkowitz, in whose office I was now sitting, began painting a different picture. "Remember what I said on the phone when you first called me, that when you see a 102 fasting number, you'd have to have a 60 on the other end to have an average of 80?" he said. "So your results show a pretty big jump up, to 165, at the half-hour mark. Then you start falling. And so look at what happens at two hours. You're down to 73."

During the test, this would have been when I began feeling sleepy, a little confused, slow to respond. If we were coworkers and I had eaten a few doughnuts or drunk two Cokes instead of the sugary goop, I might have asked you to repeat something that I should have understood. I might have seemed spaced out.

Rather than making a U-turn at the NO TRESPASSING sign, however, my blood sugar crashed through it and kept going. Three hours into the test, I had sunk to 59, a level where my brain sensed starvation, and epinephrine zapped my central nervous system like jumper cables. This is the blood sugar rescue mission, and it made me jittery, irritable, and shaky. Not that the test necessarily caught me at my nadir; this was only the lowest point actually measured. Who knows, maybe I was at 49 ten minutes before or after being at 59. The numbers on these tests may be even worse than what's captured.

"Your pancreas is responding to a fire alarm by sending all of these engines," said Dr. Berkowitz, who has a flair for colorful metaphors.

"Insulin should bring down your blood sugar just fast enough to achieve equilibrium, but it's bringing you way past that point because of your insulin resistance."

That's because it's getting a late start and then overreacting. The pancreas contains two pools of insulin. A smaller pool allows for a nearly instantaneous secretion. A bigger storage pool then replenishes it. In diabetes, the fast-acting pool seems to dry up, which may have a genetic underpinning; that could be the DNA glitch linking my father and me. So when a glucose load arrives, no insulin is forthcoming, and blood sugar skyrockets. Only then does the storage pool refill the smaller pool, leading to a delayed insulin secretion. By now, the situation seems out of control, and the pancreas overdoes the insulin. Blood sugar drops, sometimes dramatically.

If you're eating a lot of simple sugars and other carbs and not exercising—the one thing that could move the glucose into cells without insulin's help—then you're on the fast track to type 2 diabetes without that first pool. And no one, from your doctor to the ADA, is going to give you a simple heads-up to the peril you're in.

While insulin is working to lower blood sugar, the pancreas produces another hormone, called glucagon, which is designed to reverse, or at least slow, this descent. This metabolic balancing act resembles the relationship between the accelerator and brake pedals in your car. Should blood glucose drop too low, too fast, the body panics, and the adrenal glands produce a rush, designed to convert glycogen back into glucose, stat. From out of nowhere, you feel hungry, jittery, and anxious. Your heart doesn't beat like a metronome; it pounds like a jackhammer. Your muscles start quaking. Those jitters I experienced after nearly falling asleep three hours into the test? That was my body screaming "Eat or die!" as my brain's fuel-gauge needle touched E. The brain sucks up 60 percent of the body's glucose but can't produce any on its own.

Four hours into this test, my blood sugar *still* wasn't back to my starting line. I was at 80, and then 83 at five hours. I was back at what appeared to be normal, only that's still low for me; as Dr. Berkowitz was quick to note, my new normal was a prediabetic 102. "That's what your body has grown accustomed to," he said. Relative to my prevailing set point, 79, for me, now amounts to low blood sugar.

Dr. Berkowitz turned his attention to my insulin response in an effort to help me understand my ramshackle glucose control. At the start of the test, before I drank the sugary solution, my insulin stood at 6 mcU/mL. At the one-hour mark, it registered . . . 77? Perhaps even worse, at the two-hour mark, when my blood glucose was at 73, nearing hypoglycemia, my pancreas was still blasting away. Next stop for my blood glucose, the 50s.

"That's a huge outpouring of insulin," said Dr. Berkowitz. "Think about it: Your blood sugar's going maybe 50 percent higher, but your insulin levels are 10 times higher. That's like using an atomic bomb to take out a village."

The insulin level measured as part of that test isn't solely a reflection of what the pancreas secretes; the number will also be influenced by the clearance of insulin at the liver and the body's sensitivity to the hormone. Still, an insulin reading taken two hours after a glucose challenge may be the most accurate indicator of insulin resistance. Unfortunately insulin spurts of such magnitude seem to be like Miracle-Gro for diabetes, heart disease, and cancer alike—three diseases present throughout my family history, coincidentally or not.

Dr. Berkowitz theorized that glucose in flux explained my waking in the middle of the night. I had become vigilant about avoiding carbs at night, but I still worked out late. That was making a bad situation worse.

WHEN IT COMES to blood sugar, patients describe the symptoms—fatigue, absentmindedness, irritability, the jitters—all the time, but the patient and the symptoms are usually dismissed or ignored. And even those sketchy observations and that anecdotal evidence is ahead of the research.

Our instinctive response to low blood glucose is to consume sugar. But it's a false remedy, as that short-term boost also triggers another crash. There's a name for this up-and-down condition: reactive hypoglycemia.

From the moment my blood sugar had been deemed prediabetic, I had known enough not to self-medicate a crash with sugar. What's more, I had followed my low-carb diet with a rigor that surely would have placed me in the top few percent of all prediabetics. When I first started combating this killer by cutting carbs, I was feeling better than before, but I was only surveying half the battlefield. For people like me, dampening insulin isn't enough.

Dr. Berkowitz finds that the diet of someone with reactive hypoglycemia is harder to manage than the type 2 diabetic man, woman, or child who's overweight and out of shape. With them, it's pretty cut and dry. "But your situation is much more challenging," he said. "A regular low-carb diet may not work by itself because your body doesn't have good stores of glycogen. That's the challenge here."

That complexity is one of many reasons why a medically uninformed guy like my dad never stood a chance—why most people don't seem to stand a chance. Manage this condition incorrectly and the day is divided between high blood sugar and low. "Normal" is only halfway up or down the swoop of a metabolic roller coaster.

A low-carb emphasis is also important in dealing with low blood sugar, because the highs and lows play tug-of-war. Eat in a way that reduces the highs, and the lows aren't *as* low. But a low-carb diet for reactive hypoglycemia requires fine-tuning. A strict Atkins-style approach might not provide enough fuel. In my case, I would actually need to push my blood sugar up, gently, like clockwork, throughout the day.

From behind his desk, Dr. Berkowitz pointed out a few potential leaks in what I thought was an airtight diet. His advice was to decrease the time between meals, making it less than diabetics normally do. Instead of eating every three hours, I'd now be eating every two, which has the added benefit of keeping the metabolic system humming. Mind you, he wasn't telling me to increase my calories by 50 percent. He wanted me to take a meal and divide it into two or three, to be eaten a couple of hours apart.

These more frequent feedings needed more oomph than snacks, which wouldn't provide me with enough energy; yet they should have fewer calories than full meals, which could overwhelm the capacity of my metabolic system.

All of them should include lean protein and fat, replacing some carbs and slowing the absorption of those remaining. Fat also makes you feel full in a way that, say, a lean protein, such as fish, and a salad alone won't. Those carbs I did consume would almost always come from fruits and vegetables, although even some of those, the ones higher on the glycemic index, were now crossed off my shopping list.

I had been drinking a protein shake right after waking up, and Dr. Berkowitz said to keep on with that. But he told me to add some flaxseed oil, a healthy fat, to my scoop of protein powder and handful of berries. Protein powder by itself, he cautioned, could turn into glucose quickly enough to make me hypoglycemic.

Based on Dr. Berkowitz's Atkins-inspired recommendations, outlined in the Center for Balanced Health's Optimal Food Guide; materials Dr. Westman gives to his patients; other sources; and simple trial and error, I would come to view the following items as the foundation of my diet for managing reactive hypoglycemia and beating diabetes:

- Eggs (The best way to start your day, every day. I buy them fresh from one of my neighbors, and a Chilean chef friend taught me a cooking technique of his mother's invention, halfway between frying and scrambling. After breaking two eggs in the pan, move the whites around for seventy-five seconds, working around the intact yolks. Then break apart the yolks and gently mix it all together for the remaining forty-five seconds. I give the eggs a splash of cinnamon and put sliced tomatoes on the plate, too. It looks as good as it tastes. It's the one thing I've learned to cook in three and a half years, although now I want to learn more recipes.)
- Certain fruits (such as avocados, peaches, plums, apples, and cantaloupe)
- Certain vegetables (such as spinach, cucumbers, tomatoes, and celery)
- Certain nuts (such as almonds and walnuts; go easy on the cashews, which contain more than twice as many carbs as those two)

- All meat (such as turkey, chicken, and steak; exception: certain lunch meats can be packed with a lot of sugar, and they're not the healthiest option anyway)
- All fish (such as salmon, halibut, and sashimi, my favorite)
- Tuna, chicken, or egg salad (on lettuce wraps or Scandinavian Bran Crispbread)
- Soft cheeses (such as mozzarella and ricotta)
- Almond butter or cream cheese (great on celery for a snack!)
- Cottage cheese (spice it up with walnuts and cinnamon)
- Hummus (spread it on sliced cucumbers for a yummy snack)
- Herbal teas (with or without a packet of artificial sweetener)
- Coffee (with a nice splash of heavy whipping cream and no sweetener)
- Diet sodas (my favorites: Diet Coke Cherry and Coca-Cola Zero)
- Red wine (white wine, less frequently and in smaller amounts)
- Ultra-low-carb beer (my favorite: Michelob Ultra, especially on draft)
- Low- or no-carb protein powder (my favorites: Isopure and Metabolic Drive)

Avocado may give eggs a run for their money as the king of all antidiabetes foods. First, the measurements: 22 grams of very healthy fats, 3 grams of protein, and 13 grams of carbs, 10 of which are fiber! The single gram of sugar it contains, mannoheptulose, has a unique chemical structure that actually helps clear glucose from the blood. Rats fed a concentrated form as part of a study became more insulin sensitive. No wonder they lived 30 percent longer than rat subjects that weren't dipping into the guacamole.

The carbs that I included in my daily meal plan would be minimal in quantity and low on the glycemic index. Basically, that meant fruit, maybe a little oatmeal before noon, and vegetables afterward. Even there, however, I was going to be a picky eater at Dr. Berkowitz's behest, a far cry from my days as an omnivorous skinny guy who could devour whatever he wanted and stay thin. "Your carbs should come from the highest-fiber sources, like dark green vegetables," he said.

All sorts of cooking oils were fine, and Dr. Berkowitz's pamphlet added this guidance on preparation: "Eat foods that are prepared in butter, wine, or real cream (i.e., scampi, sautéed, cream sauce). Make sure bread crumbs, starch, or flour is not used." If you can cook, unlike me, all sorts of delicious low-carb recipes can mimic comfort foods such as pancakes (use eggs and pork rinds) and mashed potatoes (use a head of cauliflower). Dr. Westman hands out a whole packet of these recipes; they'll make your mouth water. North Carolina pork barbecue with low-carb coleslaw and no-bake cheesecake, anyone? It makes sense to start cooking, and most of the low-carb gurus I've met relish the creative challenge of eating well and healthfully.

What did Dr. Berkowitz forbid that day? Any carb foods that weren't fruits or vegetables, basically. As my early supermarket and restaurant excursions had proven, that was about 80 percent of what I had eaten my entire life.

Dr. Berkowitz began treading on hallowed ground by recommending a ban on drinking wine. *Not on your life, doc*, was what I was thinking, but I lied and told him I'd give it some thought. I already had investigated its effects on blood sugar myself, and I had concluded that a glass or two a day wouldn't pose any metabolic problems.

I had the same reaction to his admonition regarding coffee drinking, another enjoyable low-carb beverage—no-carb when consumed black— that had helped me keep my dietary sanity for more than a year. Sure, coffee may stimulate some sort of insulin and adrenal response, as Dr. Berkowitz suggested. But accented with cream after dinner, coffee had become my surrogate for cherry pie or chocolate cake.

In fact, when I thought back, I wondered if my cue to reach for that cup of coffee was more than the normal need for a quick pick-me-up. Was I also using it to medicate my blood sugar crashes? As it turns out, there is *some* sort of connection between caffeine and hypoglycemia. Studies have found that caffeine heightens the perception of the adrenal hormones as they kick in against this drop in blood sugar. Caffeine also stimulates the release of epinephrine, a fight-or-flight hormone. "Epinephrine is responsible for mobilizing energy, in the forms of glucose and free fatty acids, for imminent physical exertion," says Kevin J. Acheson, Ph.D., a researcher in the nutrition and health department of the Nestlé Research Center in Lausanne, Switzerland. "If physical activity doesn't ensue, all those circulating free fatty acids interfere with glucose uptake by the muscle."

That might explain why researchers see higher glucose levels in the blood of those who recently ingested caffeine. And *that*, in turn, might explain what researchers usually find when they study caffeine's short-term effect on blood sugar: reductions in both glucose tolerance and insulin sensitivity. For diabetics, that would seem doubly bad.

Not so fast, though. Epidemiological studies, which have a much longer time horizon, find that people who drink six or seven or more cups of coffee a day—about twice what the average American drinks—have a 50 percent lower chance of developing diabetes than those who drink only a few cups a day or less. This despite the tendency of heavy coffee drinkers to engage in unhealthy behaviors such as smoking cigarettes, eating poorly, and gaining excess weight.

There are several possible explanations for what seems like a contradiction. For one, the guinea pigs in studies of caffeine's short-term effects have tended to be younger individuals who don't suffer from glucose intolerance, excessive insulin production, or diabetes. And while caffeine and coffee aren't as different from each other as apples and oranges, they're not interchangeable. Caffeine is a pure molecule, and as such its effects can be easily identified. Coffee contains more than a hundred biologically active plant chemicals, including a parade of disease-fighting antioxidants. Inflammation is a hallmark of type 2 diabetes. Perhaps those antioxidants help neutralize it.

What's more, extrapolating the results of short-term studies over the longer term is risky, since other factors can intervene over time—although, at least in the case of these studies, the unhealthy lifestyle factors that tended to accompany heavy coffee drinking should have further increased, not diminished, the odds of becoming diabetic. Caffeine does, however, raise energy expenditure and fat burning. Over time, the effect this has on body weight could help prevent diabetes.

Finally, while the initial effects of caffeine on the human body can be acute, over time the body adapts. It only takes blood pressure and heart rate five days to adapt completely to caffeine's effects, so glucose metabolism might have a similar timeline. This might explain why the acute effects seem to wash out in long-term studies.

So while you can debate whether coffee or caffeine helps those with insulin resistance, it doesn't appear to hurt them, on balance.

In closing, Dr. Berkowitz tweaked my supplement stack by adding a probiotic, acidophilus, to be taken before breakfast and dinner, as well as a 100-milligram daily dose of CoQ10. This nutrient purportedly boosts energy by making muscle cells more efficient at using the oxygen delivered by the bloodstream.

Above all, my new doctor emphasized the need for consistency. This, he said, was of paramount importance. All it would take was one missed or one carb-loaded meal to throw my blood sugar out of whack. My body would spend the rest of the day playing catch-up, and if my glucose-tolerance test offered any indication, my body would lose.

DR. BERKOWITZ USES the analogy of filling up an automobile at the pump in describing reactive hypoglycemia and thin diabetics. Having been topped off, the car should have more energy, not less, than before. But when people with reactive hyperglycemia top off with carbs, their energy drops shortly thereafter. Dr. Berkowitz likens it to pouring gas into a tank, only to find that the tank has a hole in the bottom. Their body burns through carbs at a highly accelerated rate. Call it metabolic overdrive.

It sounds counterintuitive, but Dr. Berkowitz sees some overweight patients whose metabolism zooms. As for me, my body burns through glucose so rapidly that the blood sugar–insulin seesaw slams up and down several times a day, unless I strategize to prevent it. "Dropping like that is not normal," says Dr. Berkowitz of my blood sugar's reaction to the test. "I think it's a big problem in our society," he says. "I take that back. I think it's a huge problem. It's being missed because no one's looking for it." One reason that doctors aren't looking for reactive hypoglycemia is that thinness makes for a brilliant disguise. "When you're thin, doctors usually assume you're healthy and then downplay your complaints," he says.

The question is whether this chronic *hypo*glycemia leads to the chronic *hyper*glycemia of type 2 diabetes. In other words, is it prediabetes? On the fourth day of the ADA conference in New Orleans, a debate was held to answer a related question: "Is there a distinct entity called prediabetes?" The "pro" argument was put forth by one of the world's leading diabetes experts, Dr. Tuomilehto of the University of Helsinki. The expert putting forth the "con" argument was Nicholas J. Wareham, M.B., Ph.D., F.R.C.P., director of the Medical Research Council Epidemiology Unit and codirector of the Institute of Metabolic Science in Cambridge, England.

It was a spirited debate by two very smart men. At the end of Dr. Tuomilehto's presentation, an audience member stepped to a microphone in the aisle and voiced a paradox that many doctors confront: "I have two patients. Patient A is a lean person, his fasting sugar is 106, and when I did a glucose-tolerance test, his one-hour was 218 and his two-hour, 165. He has no family members with a history of diabetes. He's lean and athletic. I did an A1C and he had a 5.8. Patient B is obese with high cholesterol and hypertension, and both of his parents have type 2 diabetes. His fasting sugar is 75 and his A1C is 5.2. Which of the two patients is more prediabetic and what should I do?"

Dr. Tuomilehto felt that the second patient would be at higher risk based on typical risk-scoring systems for diabetes—meaning, check a box if you're overweight, another if diabetes runs in your family, and so on. He had little to add beyond that. This question was being posed by a doctor and answered by a leading diabetes expert in an exhibit hall containing dozens, if not hundreds, of other diabetes experts as part of the world's preeminent diabetes conference. Yet it didn't seem to occur to anyone that Patient A must be frequently and severely hypoglycemic to have 200-plus blood sugars and a nearly normal A1C. What's more, the doctor's question wasn't a question. Based on his two-hour glucose-tolerance test score alone, the thin patient isn't at risk of becoming diabetic.

By definition, he already is.

· · ·

DR. VERNON HAS a name for that doctor's thin patient, and for me. According to her, we are metabolically obese, normal-weight individuals— fat men inhabiting thin bodies. "There used to be this simplistic notion that if you're thin, you're okay; and if you're fat, you're not," she says. "Well, there are people who are thin and yet metabolically unhealthy. They can have a vascular disease that's linked to an insulin problem, not to a fat problem."

The liver reacts to a person's metabolic state by storing resources or spending them. High insulin levels cause it to shift completely toward storage, in part by turning off fat burning. "The thinking used to be, 'Weight's the problem, so if you take off the weight, your metabolism gets fixed,'" she says. "It turns out that's not true."

Fair enough, but my pancreas secretes ten times more insulin than it should, and I'm rail thin. "Not all fat cells gather or release fat at the same rate," says Dr. Vernon. "You can be one of those people who shifts toward the storage side even though you're not accumulating fat." When my blood sugar is too low, my cells, including the ones in my brain, are starved for energy. Eventually the liver runs out of its reserves, too. So my body starts cannibalizing the protein in my muscle tissue.

"This is why reactive hypoglycemia is an issue if you're a guy trying to bulk up by adding some muscle mass," says Dr. Vernon. "You're tearing down what you're making. What you need to do is eat enough protein to gain lean body mass and eat mostly fat the rest of the time. 'Cause fat won't trigger that up-and-down thing."

No wonder metabolically messed-up guys like me thud our heads on our desks in the afternoon. The brain is a fuel hog. Hypoglycemia starves the organ, which explains my headaches. We also become forgetful, anxious, aggressive, moody, tired, and unable to concentrate. When blood glucose drops to unsafe levels, the body must save its CPU. And when the brain needs something, well, the biceps or quads will just have to wait.

The LoBAG experiments also offer provocative insight into how the nonobese might develop type 2 diabetes. If a dietary shift to low carbs improves glucose metabolism without any attendant drop in body weight, might high carbs degrade glucose metabolism even in someone who doesn't experience any weight gain as a result?

I posed that question to one of the researchers behind those experiments, the University of Minnesota's Mary C. Gannon, Ph.D. *"If* a person with type 2 diabetes has been on our LoBAG diet and has seen an improvement in A1C without weight loss; and *if* he or she goes back to a higher-carb [55 percent] diet, the A1C increases without weight gain," she responded. "This was demonstrated in our studies. So in a highly controlled situation, the answer to your question is yes." She further qualified her answer by noting that all of the type-2 diabetics in the study could still secrete insulin. When we e-mailed, she hadn't completed a study using type 2 diabetics taking medication to control their blood glucose. This should add further insight.

Given the consequences of ignoring reactive hypoglycemia, the way my father did, the question becomes: How do you spot it in yourself, given its stealth? According to Dr. Berkowitz, a glucose-tolerance test can reveal information that strongly suggests reactive hypoglycemia:

- Any drop of more than 30 mg/dL within one hour.
- A half-hour, one-hour, or two-hour reading lower than your fasting measurement.
- A significantly lower A1C compared with fasting blood glucose.

He adds that a flat curve where the blood sugar does not rise significantly (less than 20 mg/dL) is also consistent with another mysterious strain of hypoglycemia.

CASSANDRA FORSYTHE, PH.D., knows what it's like to do everything right but feel as if your energy is slipping away by the moment. But with a rippling six-pack and a 135-pound bench for four sets, she is hardly a neurotic housewife, which is how doctors once labeled women with chronic hypoglycemia. In fact, calling her that might put your own health at risk. Especially if she hasn't eaten within the past few hours, in which case you might find yourself being smacked with a twenty-five-pound dumbbell.

The pretty twenty-nine-year-old is equally serious about what she puts into her body. In May 2009 she received her doctorate in kinesiology from the University of Connecticut in Storrs. Forsythe also served a yearlong internship in the local school system en route to becoming a registered dietitian. She is also the author of *Perfect Body Diet* and the coauthor of *The New Rules of Lifting for Women*.

I'm thinking to myself that she could have been the first book's cover model, were she so inclined, when she confirms that it was discussed, although her dissertation stood in the way. When she was still living in her hometown of Prince George, British Columbia, she would rack up wins at small-town swimsuit contests. "Ben Affleck saw me in a bikini!" she says, laughing. Apparently in 1999, the actor and his costar Gary Sinise, who were in Canada filming *Reindeer Games*, went to the Iron Horse Pub, where the contest was being held. Several women planning to enter the competition, including Forsythe, had spotted the actors out for dinner a few nights earlier and invited them.

The inner workings of Forsythe's body are anything but perfect, however. She wrote her dissertation on the ideal fat composition of a low-carb diet, and much of her other academic work involved carbohydrate metabolism and diabetes. She could have written much of this work in the first person, given her own blood sugar issues.

Long before dominating the bikini circuit, Forsythe, who was adopted, was a small girl with a sweet tooth. Her cat was named Candy because on weekends young Cassandra would take her allowance and head straight for the local candy store. As if that wasn't enough sugar, her mom stocked the fridge with soda. Forsythe remembers drinking it and enduring awful headaches afterward. At the time, she didn't know why.

By her early teens, she couldn't eat candy anymore, either, at least not without feeling sick. Chronic yeast infections were among an assortment of health problems that, in hindsight, probably resulted from volatile blood sugar. So at fifteen, Cassandra, who'd always wanted to be an American Gladiator, began working at a health-food store. Naturally curious, she experimented with fish oil and other health tonics. She also began grilling doctors about what might or might not help improve her health. "In my midteens I started doing yeast-free diets, which contain no sugar and no bread," she recalls.

Despite her dietary diligence, she didn't feel like herself much of the time. "I'd feel incredibly shaky, hungry, and irritable if I went longer than three or four hours between meals," Forsythe says. "And I'd feel even hungrier after I ate certain carb foods, such as fruits." One day she was at a bar drinking a Smirnoff Ice when she blacked out. The same thing happened in the gym, after twenty minutes on the elliptical trainer. Already feeling light-headed, she sensed a chill washing over her body. She stepped off the machine and lost consciousness on a stretching mat. After coming to, she waited until her blood sugar rose so that she could buy some food.

In 2000, she took a glucose-tolerance test that recorded a nadir of 30, twice as low as my bottom number, although she didn't spike first, making the extent of her decline less than mine in absolute terms. Wanting to know the cause of hypoglycemic attacks powerful enough to knock her out, she visited several endocrinologists, none of whom could explain it. As time passed, her frustration grew.

"Do you ever watch that TV show called *Mystery Diagnosis*?" she asks me one evening over a low-carb meal at Bellini's Italian Eatery in South Windsor, Connecticut. "People have unexplained things wrong with them, and they search endlessly to figure out what's wrong. They visit all these doctors and begin thinking it's all in their head. A lot of doctors don't care that much about trying to help you. If they can't solve it by looking in your eyes and down your throat and taking a blood test, they don't care. That's how I felt, anyway."

According to various tests, she had decent-enough glucose tolerance. She wasn't even excessively insulin resistant. Still, her doctors wondered why her pancreas was an insulin geyser. A well-known endocrinologist in Connecticut, someone specializing in endocrine cancers, theorized that an insulin-secreting tumor might be crashing her blood sugar. To find out, he scheduled her for a pancreatic stimulation test.

Yeah, it's as bad as it sounds. Hearing Forsythe describe the test makes it sound like an experiment undertaken by Dr. Frankenstein. First, catheters were threaded into the artery supplying her pancreas. Another catheter was positioned in her neck, exiting the jugular vein. Doctors would stimulate insulin's release by injecting calcium into the catheter leading to her pancreas. Doctors would measure the exit rate of the solution as it was leaving the second catheter.

Forsythe spent five hours lying on a frigid table with her head cocked; it took doctors longer than normal to feed catheters into her femoral arteries because the arteries were twisted. When the experiment ended, she felt like "the worst garbage ever," to use her words. "I would not wish that procedure on my worst enemy," she says.

The doctors determined that the insulin blasts were not being caused by a pancreatic tumor. So the endocrinologist offered a medication that would make her hyperglycemic. "We want to bring your blood glucose up all the time because you're low all the time," he said.

She recalls: "I was thinking: *Are you kidding me? All you want to do is give me a drug to make my blood sugars high without discussing any dietary treatment?* I said that I wasn't going to do it. *Why did I even see this guy?* I thought. Doctors are like, 'Here's a pill and another pill and another pill.' They don't ask, 'What are you eating?' Or, 'How about trying some dietary supplements?' That's taboo, right?"

Once the tumor scenario had been ruled out, Forsythe came to realize that the solution to her hypoglycemia lay in her diet—like mine, a work in progress. A heavy dose of protein includes eggs, animal fats, and salmon. She loves vegetables and eats them whenever she can. "Peas and carrots and corn I do really well with," she says. Unlike mine, her body doesn't respond well to the natural sugar in fruit. Perhaps because she's an academic who views herself as an endlessly fascinating experiment, Forsythe is nothing if not candid and straightforward, almost clinical, when discussing her own body. Nuts have become a big part of her diet, as they are of mine, but she has irritable bowel syndrome, and nuts seem to be making it worse these days, she says. Oh well.

Forsythe's idea of a cheat day would be acetic dieting for most people, as evidenced by an incident that occurred during her internship. "It was

Mexican Fiesta Day in the elementary school system, so I designed a new menu using an apple-and-jicama salad. [A jicama is a Mexican turnip, basically.] It's so good, and I put some raisins on it because the kids like that stuff. They didn't eat it but I ate it. And there was some sugar in the apples, but just a little bit."

Her blood sugar is still low quite often. Waking up can be hard for Forsythe because after a night's sleep her blood sugar registers between 60 and 70 mg/dL. Her insulin levels barely blip on the radar screen then as well. With little insulin to push her any lower, she takes advantage by doing cardio first thing in the morning. "I'll walk the dogs and run around the field for thirty minutes and be fine," she says. "By the time I'm home, I'll want to eat. I'll have two slices of Ezekiel 4:9 bread [aka sprouted grain bread], which is high protein and low glycemic. If I weren't walking the dogs, I would just have one slice of bread to limit my carbs. I'll combine that with an egg and a whole bunch of egg whites, fresh parsley, and salsa. I'll feel great afterward."

She'll become hungry about two to two and a half hours later, which puts her on more or less the same interval schedule that I follow. ("I've tried to go three, but I can't," she says.) Most of her interstitial meals are either 100 to 120 grams of chicken with a cup of frozen mixed vegetables topped with some low-carb ketchup, or a protein shake mixed with water and a can of peas. I'm glad she likes it, but that's one low-carb recipe I won't be trying.

Lunch may consist of a big salad with "a ton of protein and a ton of vegetables," she says, with a dressing (Drew's All Natural is a favorite brand) made from either canola or olive oil. She'll munch on a Ryvita crispbread heading into her afternoon lifting session, to avoid a crash during the workout, and then she'll replenish with a protein shake afterward. After another small protein-based snack or two, dinner might consist of a five-ounce pork chop with brown rice or quinoa and cooked vegetables—perhaps some combination of green beans, brussels sprouts, cauliflower, and broccoli.

Her supplement stack, like mine, is designed primarily to help steady her blood sugar. Whereas I take fish oil tablets, she takes a tablespoon or two straight from the bottle. "I was just getting sick of taking those pills," she says. She takes turmeric, and I do as well, although I use it because studies show it can help prevent prostate cancer. She takes a calcium/magnesium combo pill and vitamin D because she's lactose intolerant. Then she takes a stand-alone magnesium supplement for even more firepower. For whatever reason, people with a dysfunctional metabolic system often have low levels of this mineral when tested. She rounds out her stack with digestive enzymes and fenugreek, although I would question using the latter, given that her problem is hypoglycemia. This mainstay in ayurvedic medicine seems to lower blood sugar by stimulating the secretion of insulin, and that strikes me as fighting the wrong battle in her case.

Like me, she trains nearly every day. Were she to do cardio later in the day, when her insulin levels tend to be higher, it would speed her into hypoglycemia—hence the canine cardio. Weight training doesn't provoke the same response, so she can lift in the evening. Even then, a mere ten-minute warm-up on the treadmill will pull the rug out from under her blood sugar, forcing her to stop. "I could never run a marathon," she says, laughing.

I ask Forsythe how she feels during descents into hypoglycemia that sound more severe than mine. "When I'm falling, I get really mad at people," she says. "I think it's because adrenaline is kicking in. I try to tell them, 'I really don't mean to be like this, but you have to let me go eat something. Go away.'"

When we met for dinner, she was a newlywed, and her husband has already learned to anticipate such episodes. "When I come home from the gym and haven't eaten yet, I'm like a bear, a really mean bear, and he's like, 'Please eat something before you talk to me.' I'm like, 'Okay,' and then I eat and we're all good."

Near the end of our interview, I'm curious as to whether diabetes, or at least hypoglycemia, is a crack that extends through her family tree, like it does mine. As the question parts my lips, I remember her saying she was adopted. It turns out that when Forsythe was nineteen, she did track down her birth mother. "She has exactly the same blood sugar problems that I do," says Forsythe. "Exactly." So does a half sister.

When it comes to blood sugar, doctors are like Manhattan tourists, transfixed by what looms above. In contrast, hypoglycemia, or low blood sugar, is dark, mysterious, subterranean—and usually ignored. In Forsythe's case, the drops turned her life upside down until she had exhausted all the traditional avenues and figured things out for herself. In my case, the drops were the net result of a malfunctioning pancreas, and hence a preamble to type 2 diabetes. If you feel these same symptoms, don't be satisfied with a doctor telling you it's all in your head. Ask for a glucose-tolerance test and find out what's really going on inside your body.

13

BARELY A SHADOW CAST

Whereas most conferences send attendees home with bags of goodies, at the ADA's version, a beautiful blond lab tech is taking blood samples. Actually, it's only a prick to my left index finger at the booth of Bayer Diabetes Care, part of health care giant Bayer AG. The company knows a thing or two about blood sugar dipsticks, having offered the first-ever personal glucose meter in 1969. Thankfully, while demand for readings has mushroomed since then, the technology has shrunk. The Ames Reflectance Meter weighed more than two and a half pounds when it came out some forty years ago; most of today's models are smaller and less obtrusive than a smart phone.

Meters take a snapshot of where blood sugar stands at a given instant. But here, Bayer was debuting the first-ever A1C test that can be done at home without having to send the sample off to a lab. Results take only five minutes.

The A1C had been the headliner at an ADA press briefing held the first day of the conference. An international expert committee assembled by the ADA and two other big-time diabetes organizations had recommended adoption of the A1C as the preferred assay for diagnosing type 2 diabetes. The committee also suggested that a score of 6.5 or greater demarcates diabetes, a number below the prevailing cutoff (7.0). Were the ADA to adopt this as its new standard, it would be the first major diagnostic shift in diabetes in nearly thirty years.

Seated at the podium was the committee chairman, David N. Nathan, M.D., who is a professor of medicine at Harvard Medical School in Boston and the director of the diabetes center at Massachusetts General Hospital. The committee comprised twenty-one experts from around the globe, spanning the worlds of clinical medicine, clinical research, epidemiology, statistics, and clinical chemistry. Next to Dr. Nathan sat R. Paul Robertson, M.D., the ADA's president of medicine and science, and professor of medicine at the University of Washington in Seattle. He was there to offer comment on behalf of the ADA.

From the dais, Dr. Nathan explained that A1C, a composite measure, offers more information than any single value. After reviewing numerous clinical chemistry studies, the committee also concluded that A1C was more accurate than other measures. This assay correlates very closely with the risk of developing diabetic retinopathy (blood-vessel damage in the eyes), he continued, adding that this condition has proven to be the best proxy for long-term complications from type 2 diabetes. He mentioned ease of use as an additional advantage of the test. Overnight fasting isn't required, and it doesn't matter if the patient stopped at Dunkin' Donuts en route to the doctor's office. The A1C test doesn't cost much to administer, either.

The response of the ADA's executive committee to the findings, as relayed by Dr. Robertson, was "to support the conclusion in the paper that the A1C measurement is appropriate for diagnosing diabetes." On December 31, the ADA would amend its clinical practice guidelines to include an A1C score of 6.5 percent or higher as a fourth diagnostic indicator of diabetes, joining the preexisting thresholds for the fasting and random plasma glucose tests and the glucose-tolerance test.

I had spoken with ADA spokesman Dr. Deeb back when I first

encountered my own blood sugar problems. He had said that A1C is useful, although his explanation of why suggested a particular treatment orientation. "I see people all the time whose fasting blood sugar is 145 and whose A1C is 6.8," he had said. "That's diabetes. They get the message, go on some medicine, come back, and their A1C comes back 5.5. I pat them on the back and tell them they're taking great care of themselves, and they are. Absolutely."

Averages are a funny thing. Math was my worst subject in high school, but I know that while 7 and 5 average out to 6, so do 10 and 2. Listening to Dr. Nathan speak, I thought of my own experience. I also recalled a conversation about A1C that I'd had a year earlier with Braun, the University of Massachusetts professor whose son, Samson, is a type 1 diabetic. "I didn't realize this until I had to take care of someone with type 1 diabetes, but you can arrive at a normal A1C by so many different routes," Braun had told me on campus. "My son's doctors will be like, 'Look, his A1C is 6.3!' I'm like, 'Yeah, that's great, but last week he was over 300 four times and under 50 four times. The average is perfect, and yet a single glucose value is seldom good."

Type 2s may not have the potential to swing quite as wildly as type 1s, who can soar or plunge from the wrong insulin dose. Nonetheless, many type 2s have highly volatile blood sugar. A glucose-tolerance test is given to at-risk patients to quantify those swings. That's what told me what was going on inside my body. The A1C score? That was nothing more than a head fake in my case.

I asked Dr. Nathan a question from the audience, namely, were effects of blood sugar volatility on A1C a concern or even a consideration during the committee's deliberations? After all, suggesting a new primary diagnostic tool for type 2 diabetes has profound implications for hundreds of millions of diabetics and prospective diabetics, given ADA's global influence. "It turns out that in the nondiabetic, untreated population, hypoglycemia that would affect A1C is extraordinarily rare," answered Dr. Nathan, who moments before had emphasized that the risk for developing diabetes is a continuum, meaning there's no single line in the sand. "So in the population you're screening to see if they have a diabetic A1C, low blood sugar would virtually never play a clinically important role in affecting or perturbing that marker. I don't think it would interfere with it at all."

Except that along that continuum, blood sugar swings can become their most frenetic between the times when you're "normal" and diabetic, the metabolic purgatory labeled prediabetes. Glucose metabolism has begun malfunctioning, but like a dying man trying to fight off an attacker, the pancreas can still produce wild surges when provoked by carbs. However, because cells are now resistant to insulin's overtures, the pancreas keeps on secreting. Before the pancreatic beta cells give up the fight altogether and cease to function, insulin can turn blood sugar skyrockets into equally spectacular crashes. Tell anyone who feels extremely tired after eating a carb-packed lunch that hypoglycemia among nondiabetics (not yet, anyway) is extraordinarily rare.

As for me, five minutes after Bayer's lab tech pricked my finger in the exhibit hall, I was handed a sheet of paper listing my results. My A1C score was 5. According to that measurement, my blood sugar works perfectly well.

OF COURSE, I already knew that giving my blood sugar a perfect score based on a composite was like gluing together a hundred shards of glass and deeming that a broken mirror was in mint condition. Luckily, taking the glucose-tolerance test at Dr. Berkowitz's behest had allowed me to see the truth behind the illusion. Awareness trumped ignorance, even if managing reactive hypoglycemia would be a lifelong challenge. "The enemy you know" and all those other clichés. But I wondered: Was this medical anomaly limited to my bloodline and few others, or was it part of a bigger problem? Dr. Berkowitz is one of a small-but-growing group of physicians who think that reactive hypoglycemia might be the biggest undiagnosed health problem in America.

Dr. Berkowitz had advised me to set my sights low when looking for work on reactive hypoglycemia in the academic literature. He was right. Not much has been published, at least not recently. Strangely, though, the farther back I dug, the more information I found, and the more enlightening it became.

It's part of a trend in our country's maddening history of diabetes misguidance: Someone actually figured out reactive hypoglycemia at the turn of the century—the *twentieth* century, that is—only to be treated like a pariah rather than a prophet. His name was Seale Harris, and he was born in Cedartown, Georgia, in 1870. He received his medical degree in 1894 from the University of Virginia Medical School, undertook postgraduate work at Johns Hopkins University, and became a professor of clinical medicine at the Medical College of Alabama in Mobile. He was commissioned as a major in the U.S. Army and then decorated for his service during World War I. By 1924, he was working at the same lab bench as insulin's discoverers. Yet the first stabs at administering this miracle elixir were an art, not a science. Patients often received too much or too little. And too much at once could do more than lower high blood sugar; it could push someone too far the other way, from hyperglycemia to hypoglycemia.

Further, Dr. Harris noticed that some nondiabetics, after they ate, experienced a reaction similar to type 1s who had overdone their insulin shots—they crashed. He christened the condition hyperinsulinism, or too much ("hyper") insulin production. He had the foresight to realize that at the start of type 2 diabetes, the body produces too much insulin, not too little. Only later in the disease does production of the hormone plummet, as the beta cells of the pancreas burn out. Imagine a baseball pitcher throwing three hundred pitches every start instead of a hundred. Eventually his arm would go dead.

Dr. Harris was a dilettante, writing articles in medical journals but also hammering out biographies of other medical figures (Banting, his colleague; and J. Marion Sims, a controversial gynecologist), as well as musings on grizzly bears, temperance, and the state of the Democratic Party under President Harry S. Truman. But he was no crackpot. So prolific, eclectic, and important were his accomplishments that he earned the nickname "the Benjamin Franklin of medicine." He founded a noted diabetes clinic that would come to bear his name. Dr. Harris also held the presidency of several major medical associations. But his discovery of reactive hypoglycemia was his medical masterpiece.

Dr. Harris identified pancreatic tumors as the cause of selected hyperinsulinism cases. But he also figured out that by attributing all hypoglycemia to a rare form of tumor, medical science was missing another problem altogether. He gave this counterpart to diabetes mellitus the name reactive hypoglycemia, although others called it Harris Syndrome. He then went on to categorize five different variations of the condition. "The low blood sugar of today is the diabetes of tomorrow," wrote Dr. Harris. In stark contrast to the attitude of today's experts toward reactive hypoglycemia—"Hey, it's no problem!"—Dr. Harris was predicting the dissolution of my father's health before my father was even born.

To Dr. Harris, the solution for hyperinsulinism and the low blood sugar that it produced was eating a low-sugar diet and small, frequent meals, rather than calorie-laden two- or three-a-days. Some wealthy Europeans, at least, eyed his method with great interest; many trekked to his Alabama clinic in search of his blood sugar–mending magic. Dr. Harris's discovery received a gold star of sorts when the American Medical Association awarded him its highest honor, the Distinguished Service Medal, in 1949, nine years before he passed away.

Problem solved.

SOLUTION REJECTED. WHY was Dr. Harris's medical masterpiece packed up and stuffed in the attic for decades? Wrote author William Dufty in his lively 1975 book *Sugar Blues*: "Predictably, the medical profession landed on Dr. Harris like a ton of bricks. When his findings were not attacked, they were ignored. His discoveries, if allowed to leak out, might make trouble for surgeons, psychoanalysts, and other medical specialists." No one stood to become rich from such a commonsense, do-it-yourself solution, whereas a drug-taking diabetic becomes an annuity of sorts.

Having medical power brokers ignore the solution from the get-go assured that the prevalence of reactive hypoglycemia would only increase. It had many allies, as American consumers became enslaved by convenient carbs shoveled into a white bag and handed to them by pimple-faced teenagers wearing crooked paper hats. Harris's low-sugar diet was crushed under the tire treads of drive-through dining. In 1963, the United States had 9,474 "refreshment places" (the Bureau of the Census's label for fast-food joints before 1997) and $381 million in sales. According to recently released preliminary data for 2007, 209,819 limited-service establishments (the new term) registered $152 billion in sales.

Because reactive hypoglycemia both resulted from and reflected these trends, for patients it could become a diagnostic Rorschach test, capable of accommodating a whole host of ailments both physical (ulcers, chronic fatigue, joint pain, soft-tissue soreness, etc.) and psychological (depression, insomnia, neurosis, etc.). It was even blamed for aberrant behaviors such as criminality and addictions such as alcoholism. An otherwise insightful and prescient book from 1951, *Body, Mind and Sugar*, went so far as to blame low blood sugar "for the moral breakdown that underlies all delinquency and crime." Demand was brisk enough to prompt several dozen printings.

No doubt some of these symptoms were real, some imagined, and it was hard for doctors and patients alike to distill fact from fiction. But the plasticity of reactive hypoglycemia made many health pros skeptical of an ailment capable of accommodating such far-flung symptoms. Interestingly, those patients whose blood sugar tests have revealed legitimate reactive hypoglycemia have shown a tendency for hypochondria on personality tests, such as the Minnesota Multiphasic Personality Inventory. Then again, maybe people whose blood sugar slams up and down several times a day feel really lousy and don't know why.

Consider a case study I stumbled upon in a 1965 issue of the *Canadian Medical Association Journal*. Two doctors were describing a forty-one-year-old veteran turned salesman who had come to Westminster Hospital in London, Ontario, in 1962. The man complained of headaches, especially in the morning, before breakfast. He also experienced chest pain, leg numbness, and behavioral problems that had cost him his job and landed him in psychotherapy. This must not have worked very well, because he tried to kill himself in 1956. He reported to his new doctors that his diet was loaded up with sugary foods, potatoes, and breads, not to mention a cup of coffee heaped with sugar every few hours—perfectly (but unwittingly) timed to help push him out of a blood sugar crash, and set him up for another one. The bad habits that people can't break are usually developed for good reason. They're not inevitable. They have a context.

A thorough medical examination failed to reveal a disease that might account for this poor fellow's unraveling. As part of the exam, his fasting blood sugars ranged from 69 to 84 mg/dL—readings that would earn him a clean bill of metabolic health from most doctors today (and numbers that I would love to have). But these Canadian doctors wanted to investigate his carbohydrate metabolism with a glucose-tolerance test. After swilling his sugar drink, the man's blood sugar rose from 76 to 200 in an hour. He fell from there but was still high at the two-hour mark. His blood sugar descended into the 40s at the fourth hour before crawling back up.

During his relatively brief stay down in the 40s, he exhibited the sort of anxiety and agitation that had characterized his mental instability in adulthood. It may not have been his fault. Act crazy for a stretch every three hours or so and people start thinking you're nuts. As I heard one diabetes expert explain, it was hard to tell the drunks from the diabetics back when there were no meters in hospitals. Even today, when type 1 diabetic teens dip unaware into hypoglycemia, they're often assumed to be substance abusers. Well, type 2s and prediabetics also crash.

"This case emphasizes the fact that diabetes mellitus should always be suspected in patients with symptoms of postprandial [i.e., postmeal] hypoglycemia, especially if there is a history or evidence of familial diabetes," wrote the two doctors.

The prescription they handed the tormented man was . . . a new food-shopping list.

While the mainstream diabetes movement largely shunned Dr. Harris's views on reactive hypoglycemia, I was surprised to find such case studies when I sifted through the literature. These selected physicians had a firm grasp of a dangerous condition and offered patients a lifeline. Stumbling upon their long-forgotten words while poring through hundreds of old studies reminded me of listening to Drs. Vernon and Berkowitz and a handful of others who still see the same problem week after week in their clinics. They may not have all the answers, but to their credit, they aren't satisfied to send patients off to a diabetic destiny. They analyze the problem using their wits, gut instincts, research, and clinical experience, rather than relying on whatever dogma some higher authority has handed down to them.

I found the closest analogue to my own experience in a 1971 issue of a journal called *California Medicine*, which was renamed the *Western Journal of Medicine* in 1974, before becoming defunct in 2002. The piece amounted to an edited transcript of doctors at the University of California at San Francisco comparing notes during a weekly staff meeting. They discussed what one doctor referred to as "an interesting disorder of carbohydrate homeostasis—hypoglycemia." The patient was a twenty-six-year-old Caucasian woman who had endured headaches for six years and sought help because they had become severe. The pain would start in her neck, creep up, and wrap around her head. At peculiar times, sleepiness, chills, and tremors would wash over her. The doctors X-rayed her chest and skull, tested the electrical activity of her heart with an electrocardiogram, and analyzed her urine and blood. All came back normal.

Unlike many of today's doctors, however, hers weren't content to chalk up her state to the stresses of modern life and usher her out the door with a dose of condescension. Instead the woman underwent a glucose-tolerance test. Her blood sugar soared from 92 at the start of the test to 200 at the half-hour mark. At two hours, she was back to 100; and, at three hours, she was at 52. Reading this woman's curve, I might as well have been reading my own. Her symptoms, especially the headaches, also mimicked mine. (Remember the "band of pain" clamping around my head when I arrived at the offices of *Men's Health* in 2006?) "Reactive hypoglycemia was diagnosed and the patient was discharged with a prescription of a high-protein, low-carbohydrate diet," said Norman C. Coleman, M.D., assistant resident in medicine. "On this dietary regime she has been asymptomatic for two months since discharge from the hospital."

Later in the meeting, another doc, John H. Karam, M.D., assistant
professor of medicine, had this to say: "In an accelerated hyperinsulinism with early hypoglycemia [the woman's and my pathology] . . . the
patient is offered small, frequent, high-protein feedings which contain
no processed sugar and only limited carbohydrate."

REACTIVE HYPOGLYCEMIA ENJOYED a brief renaissance in the
early 1970s, around the time the study of the twenty-six-year-old was
written up. The condition became fodder for academic journals and
mainstream magazines (*Vogue*, etc.) alike. (If it were today, *Star* magazine and *Extra!* would no doubt be devoting twenty-word blurbs or
twenty-second sound bites to some actress sending a Twitter update
about her low blood sugar.) None other than *Consumer Reports* set aside
motor vehicle and washing-machine reviews to attempt an adjudication
of the matter in a 1971 piece titled "Low-Blood Sugar: Fact or Fiction?"
Much of this fairly skeptical piece focused on quacks hawking glandu-
lar extracts from animals as surrogates for what some shady doctors had
diagnosed as burned-out adrenal glands in hypoglycemic patients. But
the article's overarching verdict was that reactive hypoglycemia, dubbed
"functional" hypoglycemia by the author, was real and could be managed by decreasing sugar and starch intake and eating smaller, more
frequent meals. Which is great advice.

One other sentence caught my eye: "Functional hypoglycemia is
likely to occur in people with a family history of diabetes mellitus and
may be a forerunner, by several years, of that disease."

After this flurry of coverage, the condition disappeared again from
doctors' radar screens. Too bad it didn't disappear from patients' bodies. A fad may have come and gone, but America's blood sugar roller-
coaster ride didn't just continue apace. It ratcheted up a gear. Exactly
how many people are walking around with normal A1C scores and reactive hypoglycemia is hard to tell. After all, no one's looking for them or
doing the necessary tests because they tend to be normal weight or thin,
and thought not to be at risk.

Someone like Dr. Vernon, who knows the telltale signs, encounters them all the time in the heartland. "Yesterday, I saw a lanky guy in the emergency room of the hospital, and he had a leg wound," she says. "This was a classic Kansas farmer. I know the mind-set: *I have to harvest, honey. Just put duct tape on it.* But he had chainsawed a big ol' gaping hole in his leg! He was cutting hedge, which is a really tough wood, and it kicked back against him.

"I examined the wound, looked at him, and said, 'My God, didn't this *hurt?'* Usually when you chainsaw your leg, you can feel it.

"He's like, 'Well . . . it kind of burned a little.'

"This guy had bad diabetic neuropathy, he had no clue, and nobody had figured it out. He didn't even want any pain medicine before he went in for surgery!"

If that farmer can't feel a chain saw, it's easier to understand how diabetics miss infections of the feet and legs until a doctor is wielding a different saw. That's one reason why diabetic amputations are so rampant.

Are the numbers for reactive hypoglycemia hard to track because the condition is rare, as suggested by organizations such as the ADA and The Endocrine Society? Or is it hard to quantify because it's so common? I have it. My editor on the *Men's Health* feature, Adam Campbell, a very fit-looking guy in his thirties, has it. You may have it, too. A lot of people just don't feel well a lot of the time. Their fasting glucose level is relatively normal. Their A1C is A-OK. Yet their bodies sputter.

The rapid rise of a condition such as polycystic ovary syndrome may offer clues to reactive hypoglycemia's prevalence, since they share the same metabolic underpinning. Estimates are that 10 to 20 percent of child-bearing-age women in the United States suffer from PCOS. The prevailing theory is that in millions of women insulin resistance leads to overproduction. Women naturally produce very small amounts of male hormones, but the excessive insulin ups their production. Often the result is menstrual problems, ovarian cysts, and in many cases, diminished fertility. What's scary is that our high-sugar meals and increasingly stressful lives are exactly the one-two punch needed for reactive hypoglycemia to skyrocket. If it hasn't already, this trend has the potential to create a whole new class of diabetics, the outwardly fit-looking, inwardly ill. Diabetes has always been a disease of the overweight, but it's morphing into something additional now.

When I did a phone interview with Dr. Vernon, a family physician, before visiting her in Kansas, she profiled the following patients. Notice how different they are, yet how predictable the underlying progression becomes:

- A twenty-year-old Hawaiian kid who weighs 238 pounds and has a BMI of 35, which is obese. His fasting glucose is 94 and his fasting insulin is 9.4, both of which are on the high side but still normal. One hour into a glucose-tolerance test, his insulin hits 100. At three hours, his blood sugar is down to 74. Too much insulin equals low blood sugar.
- A fifty-year-old redhead who comes in because she's a bit overweight. Her fasting glucose is a prediabetic 115, but the sugar goop shoots her up to a very diabetic 261, at which point her insulin is blasting away at 119. At three hours, her blood sugar has fallen to 41. Too much insulin came too late. Her glucose and insulin curves should be finely calibrated; instead, they're totally out of sync.
- A 269-pound vegetarian woman who showed up with a prediabetic fasting glucose of 123. At two hours, her blood sugar is at 200, and her insulin is 632—off the charts. "When I pitch this slide in front of docs, I say, 'Who needs to hire a bacteria to make insulin in the laboratory? You can just use this lady's pancreas.' She should have a career." Only she'll never be able to sustain this outpouring. Drugs will have to pick up the slack unless she takes action.

"Lest you think that all I ever do is just gather information, not ever fix anybody, let's look at how she did," said Dr. Vernon, who wrote up a vegetarian low-carb diet for the woman. In three months, she lost twenty-five pounds, her fasting glucose dropped below 100, and many of her other markers of metabolic syndrome normalized.

Many of her other patients achieved similarly impressive results.

Case studies can't be relied upon to prove a theory, needless to say. But our original understanding of diabetes was largely informed by case studies—the ones outlined in those accounting ledgers of Dr. Joslin's.

Ignoring this data becomes a self-fulfilling prophecy; I guarantee that we'll never know anything about the scope of reactive hypoglycemia if we never bother to look for it. Dr. Vernon and a select group of physicians like her rattle off individuals from all walks of life, in all shapes and sizes, and their data contradict this notion that carb-induced hypoglycemia is extremely rare.

What's more, while a prodigious amount of ink has been spilled about what specific number demarcates hypoglycemia, that's not the point. The huge outpourings of insulin driving blood sugar down, down, down are exceedingly unhealthy, no matter where the blood sugar happens to register at the exact moment a nurse says, "Can you roll up your sleeve, please?" What matters most is that insulin blasts are hitting 75, 100, 200—not whether someone bottoms out at 55, 58, or 67 as a result.

A DECADE INTO the twenty-first century, some of the largest organizations in the world entrusted to lead the charge against type 2 diabetes are actually heading in a different direction. When I interviewed ADA spokesman Dr. Deeb for my *Men's Health* feature, I asked him, "How much does the ADA look at hypoglycemia, specifically reactive hypoglycemia? Does it focus more on the high side?"

"It really does," he said. "Hypoglycemia is an endocrine disease. Diabetes is, too, but hypoglycemia is caused by tumors of the pancreas or other conditions that make people's blood sugar low. [Those conditions are] not truly diabetes and not dealt with by the ADA."

Guidelines on hypoglycemia published recently by The Endocrine Society rely heavily on a construct called Whipple's triad. Drawn up in the 1930s by Allen O. Whipple, who pioneered pancreatic surgery, the triad holds that hypoglycemia is real—as opposed to imaginary, I guess—when three conditions apply: (1) if hypoglycemic symptoms occur; (2) if your blood glucose reads low in tandem with those symptoms; and (3) if raising your blood glucose back to normal alleviates those symptoms.

I found myself scratching my head while reading the progressions embedded in the hypoglycemia-without-diabetes section of The Endocrine Society's guidelines. First they instruct the doctor to review the patient's medical history for anything suggesting a cause for the hypoglycemia—a tumor, a hormone deficiency, drugs, or something equally exotic. The issue of whether the patient starts his day with two jelly doughnuts and a coffee with two sugars isn't raised, however.

Assuming nothing is found, the next step is for the doctor to measure plasma glucose, insulin, and other agents "during an episode of spontaneous hypoglycemia." How would this ever occur? Your guess is as good as mine. Maybe if you *happened* to be in the office for an appointment, and you *happened* to feel hypoglycemic, a doctor could drop everything, run in, and take these measurements—which are still only one-offs, rather than a dynamic, integrated series. You want a filmstrip, not one frame. But the implication is that the lows are context-free and unpredictable as a result.

At that point, the doctor is told to attempt a re-creation of the episode using a fast of up to three days (sounds fun, huh?) or a mixed meal (finally, food is at least mentioned). The guidelines say these are "the circumstances in which symptomatic hypoglycemia is likely to occur." Only a glucose challenge would be far more likely to provoke hypoglycemia; properly mixing the macronutrients of meals prevents this from happening! In their daily lives, most people *don't* make a conscious effort to balance their meals properly. That's the problem. Hamburger bun, carbs; french fries, carbs; large soda, carbs; dessert, carbs—oh, and there's a slip of something resembling beef buried in there somewhere.

If hypoglycemia isn't documented through Whipple's triad at this point, the patient is deemed to be okay, and the process ends. If hypoglycemia is documented, the doctors are told to pursue a series of invasive, labyrinthine procedures in search of a pancreatic tumor that might be causing the problem. This is exactly the hellish process Forsythe underwent before fixing the problem by tweaking her diet.

Why would you require the presence of Whipple's triad for a diagnosis of hypoglycemia but forbid the test that seems best suited to identify it? The staggered blood draws catch something at least close to the nadir (which addresses condition number two), and the doctor administering the test should, as Dr. Berkowitz did with me, have you jot down symptoms on the half hour (which addresses condition number one). You don't really confirm condition number three until you leave the doctor's office feeling like a zombie, stumble into the nearest restaurant, order something to eat or drink, take a bite or sip, and slowly come back to life. *Oh, my blood sugar was low,* you realize.

I e-mailed the lead author, Philip E. Cryer, M.D., professor of endocrinology and metabolism at Washington University School of Medicine, and asked him about the absence of the glucose-tolerance test in this whole progression. "A glucose-tolerance test is never indicated in the evaluation of a patient for hypoglycemia," he wrote back.

That has an "end-of-story" ring to it, but that test had solved the case of at least one hypoglycemic patient: namely, me. Dr. Berkowitz had suspected reactive hypoglycemia based on the discrepancy between my A1C and my fasting blood sugar; used a glucose-tolerance test, not only to confirm his theory, but also to map out how my blood sugar and insulin interacted; and then customized my diet to smooth out all the missteps. As a result, I stopped "dropping," and I felt much better. My blood sugar profile improved rather than deteriorated. As the owner of this body, I was one happy customer. It struck me that this is how medicine should work but too often doesn't.

I probably would have accepted what Dr. Deeb and others said and left it at that were it not for my father, who lay dying from the same condition that I have, not from some pancreatic tumor. And I was staring at test results showing that carbs spiked my blood sugar to 160-plus before dropping it into the 50s. Before taking corrective action, I had felt my body was slipping from my control and into the hands of diabetes, whose grip had been tightening.

Pancreatic tumors can indeed produce fasting hypoglycemia. Even in the absence of a cue from sugar, this alien body in the pancreas can make it secrete insulin, which will drive down blood sugar for no apparent reason. But that's a fundamentally different condition from reactive hypoglycemia. In the latter case, a couple of Twinkies, not a tumor, would do the trick. Whereas someone with a pancreatic tumor has low fasting blood sugar, someone with reactive hypoglycemia, like me, tends to have high fasting blood sugar. The effect is the opposite.

Dr. Berkowitz puts it another way: "The ADA recognizes hypoglycemia when a type 1 diabetic takes too much insulin. Well, if your body is making too much insulin itself, isn't it the same thing? Common sense would dictate that."

The CDC at least recognizes reactive hypoglycemia as a condition, as does the National Institute of Diabetes and Digestive and Kidney Diseases, or NIDDK, of NIH. As for the condition's provenance, NIDDK/NIH says in a fact sheet: "The causes of most cases of reactive hypoglycemia are still open to debate. Some researchers suggest that certain people may be more sensitive to the body's normal release of the hormone epinephrine, which causes many of the symptoms of hypoglycemia. Others believe deficiencies in glucagon secretion might lead to reactive hypoglycemia."

In my case, it's not as if my *perception* of epinephrine is some sort of mirage, as the NIDDK/NIH theory is suggesting. Epinephrine is being released for a very good reason—because my blood sugar has fallen 100 points in an hour. That hormone, at least, is working properly. The maybe-your-glucagon-isn't-working argument seems equally misguided. After a plunge that steep, you can't tell me that the last 10 or 20 points of the drop occur because my glucagon isn't kicking in. That hormone is simply trying to brake a roller coaster clattering downhill. It's just over-matched.

NIDDK/NIH also remains unconvinced that carbs are the major cause: "Although some health professionals recommend a diet high in protein and low in carbohydrates, studies have not proven the effectiveness of this kind of diet to treat reactive hypoglycemia," says the same backgrounder.

While the sheet recommends protein foods, fruits and vegetables, and dairy, it also tells those with reactive hypoglycemia to consume "starchy foods such as whole-grain bread, rice, and potatoes." Those starches will jack up a person's blood sugar faster than eating sugar with a spoon. That's the cause of the condition, not the cure. And if the jury is still out on low-carb diets, as they suggest, then why are carbs used as the triggering mechanism for a metabolic stress test? No one's being handed a protein shake or a glass of fish oil to slug down.

Granted, my hypoglycemia was induced by a drink containing 75 grams of pure sugar and nothing else. But one original-size Jamba Juice Fit N' Fruitful contains 72 grams of sugar (84 grams of carbs), and the standard recommendation of consuming 50 percent of your calories from carbohydrates translates to 250 to 300 grams' worth a day. Split over three squares a day—or two and a half, as the AAFP's Dr. King recommended to me—means consuming more than a glucose-tolerance test's worth of carbs at each meal. "We use glucose tolerance as a metabolic stress test and yet prescribe a diet that produces that at every meal," says Raab. "It highlights just how ridiculous this advice is."

EVEN THOUGH CDC and NIDDK/NIH acknowledge reactive hypoglycemia, they don't seem to view it as a public health problem. For example, neither organization collects any data on how many U.S. adults are chronically hypoglycemic, even though it's the shadowy flip side of the fastest-growing disease in the country, type 2 diabetes. What's worse, both CDC and NIDDK/NIH claim there is insufficient evidence to suggest that reactive hypoglycemia leads to diabetes, even though reactive hypoglycemia is a by-product of insulin resistance.

The AAFP has published research on reactive hypoglycemia but offers no clinical guidelines or policies that might help doctors and patients manage the condition. As for the American Dietetic Association, in their *Nutrition Care Manual*, they quote a piece in the *New England Journal of Medicine* to the effect that reactive hypoglycemia is of "non diabetic origin," and "a clinical syndrome with diverse causes." "There's no discussion of reactive hypoglycemia in the *NCM* that indicates it being a risk for type 2 diabetes," Eleese Cunningham, R.D., an ADA dietitian, wrote me.

Until a study is conducted to prove otherwise, normal-weight or even thin prediabetics such as me have to play detective. Are there two sets of people, diabetic versus nondiabetic, each with reactive hypoglycemia, traveling through life on separate tracks, headed to different destinations? Or should they be thought of as occupying the same track, but at different junctions? Under the latter scenario, the nondiabetics with reactive hypoglycemia could "catch up" with diabetics if they didn't take corrective action, and end up with the same complications, not to mention the same fate.

Unfortunately, the view that reactive hypoglycemia and type 2 diabetes are separate and distinct phenomena dominates in the current literature. Those new guidelines from The Endocrine Society are a good example. Section 2.0 is titled "Evaluation and management of hypoglycemia in persons without diabetes mellitus," and Section 3.0 is titled, "Evaluation and management of hypoglycemia in persons with diabetes mellitus."

My case shows the limitations of this rigid divide. I look at those two headings, read what lies below them, and think: *Okay, well, I'm not diabetic, but I have impaired fasting glucose and impaired glucose tolerance. So I am prediabetic. And my carb-induced rise and fall in blood sugar has been mapped out by a test—but the guidelines before me dismiss both the condition and the use of this test to diagnose the condition. Only my father had the same glucose metabolism as I do, and now he's dying from diabetes. So I should . . .*

Ignore the guidelines. In contrast to the ADA, The Endocrine Society, and others, Dr. Vernon believes the chronic rise and fall of blood sugar is a nearly inevitable part of the progression from prediabetes to full-on diabetes. Insulin resistance worsens, insulin secretions increase, and blood sugar drops become more pronounced. Losing the ability to keep blood sugar in bounds is impaired glucose tolerance. That's only a step or two away from type 2 diabetes.

AT ONE OF my last encounters at the ADA conference, I was offered a different sort of pick-me-up at the booth of Generex Biotechnology. The signage suggests the sort of biotech outfit Michael Crichton might have conjured for one of his 1980s thrillers, an effect cemented when an avuncular man wearing a business suit approaches me. With his white hair parted on the side, he's a dead ringer for the late actor Richard Widmark. His name is Gerald Bernstein, M.D., and he is the vice president of medical affairs for Generex, as well as an associate professor at Albert Einstein College of Medicine in New York City.

Historically, self-administered diabetes care has been rather barbaric, Bayer's sexy lab tech notwithstanding. You pricked yourself in the finger, measured the sugar using a meter and a strip, and then plunged an insulin-filled needle into a vein if the reading was high. Generex has developed a novel delivery vehicle that wouldn't cramp the style of a diabetic starlet in a nightclub. Oral-lyn, Generex's flagship product, allows you to spray insulin into the permeable tissues lining your mouth, a shortcut to the bloodstream.

Another fast-acting product, Glucose RapidSpray, uses the same delivery technology for a quick sugar rush. If your blood sugar falls, just squirt; to the uninitiated, it would appear as if you were freshening your breath, which you sort of are, since it comes in orange or raspberry flavors. "Don't Delay. Just Spray!" urges the packaging, which also assures fat-phobes that the spray is "fat free."

Throughout Generex's promotional literature, the message is clear: Type 2 diabetes is to be out-engineered, not out-hustled. "As quality of life improves, even slightly, a better diet and technology will lead to increased weight and less physical labor," writes Dr. Bernstein in one of the papers enclosed in a folder he hands me. "For many this will be a great benefit but along with it will be the greater expression of the genes for diabetes."

Apparently we can all look forward to a glorious future of plumpness and sloth. We'll just have to deal with this pesky little type 2 diabetes problem as a side effect.

I field a question from Dr. Bernstein when he wanders back, namely, why is someone as thin as I am interested in diabetes, anyway? I explain that, my build notwithstanding, my blood sugar slithers up and down like a snake. He tells me that going up as high as 180 isn't abnormal, even though the official cutoff point for prediabetes is 160 at the two-hour mark of a glucose-tolerance test. As for the subsequent crash, he hands me a bottle of RapidMist. Take a hit when you feel low during a workout, he says. Otherwise, according to him, I needn't worry about my blood sugar.

"There was [a] time when it was thought that reactive hypoglycemia was a precursor to diabetes, but that's largely been dismissed," says Dr. Bernstein. "It's not a problem, really. I see it all the time in patients."

Exactly.

14

DISSOLVED

At the Joslin Center, the walls of the rotunda are lined with paintings of scenes emblematic of diabetes: a cherubic young girl receiving an insulin injection from her mother; Priscilla White, the woman who pioneered treatment of gestational diabetes, exiting a car; a group of fresh-faced boys learning diabetes tips at summer camp; a dignified researcher, Alex Marble, standing before a lab full of beakers.

Another picture was commissioned, painted, and hung, but when the time came to break through a wall in the foyer to make room for a new Walgreens, this canvas was stored, hidden from view. According to Dr. Barnett, who had first insisted on including this scene in the series, "The artist painted a middle-aged women in bed with a foot frame parted, looking anxiously at her pregangrenous, dusky-colored set of toes and foot while Dr. Howard Root [a Dr. Joslin associate] and an operating room-garbed surgeon looked on." Even at Diabetes Central, where they deal with blindness and other horrible diabetes complications every day, losing a foot or limb to the disease still makes everyone queasy.

Dr. Barnett was surprised to learn that my father had lost nearly all of his leg. "Above the knee is called a Civil War amputation," he said. "They hate to do it now; they'll do it only if the leg is gangrenous. Your father may have been septic. Was he reticent about going to the doctor's office? He might have waited too long."

Several months before the operation, my father had been vacationing in Cape May, New Jersey, at a beach house rented by his brother, my Uncle Hughie. My father was asked ahead of time what he was drinking these days, and he said ginger ale. Hughie supplied his fridge accordingly. Even at this late stage, at least a decade into the disease, Hughie had no idea that his older brother was diabetic. Perhaps my father was ashamed of it for some reason. But knowing him, it was simply out of sight, out of mind, even as diabetes was devouring him. Over the weekend, my father went through several bottles of the soda, and not the carb-free version.

A few months later, Hughie could tell something was up when he called my father one day. The voice on the other end of the line sounded confused, tired, faint. Hughie barely recognized it, in fact.

"What the hell is wrong with you, Tucker?" he asked.

"I didn't tell you, but I've got diabetes, and I didn't take care of myself."

"Well, for God's sake, get to the hospital. You sound horrible."

"I don't do hospitals."

"Well, how do you feel about dying?" said Hughie, beyond exasperation.

My father didn't seek help. When Hughie phoned him a few days later, my father struggled even to speak. This time, Hughie implored him to dial 911.

"I can't get up and I don't have any strength," said my father.

Hughie then asked to speak to my father's wife. She insisted anew that my father wouldn't be willing to go to the hospital.

During a subsequent call, according to Hughie, my father passed out. Apparently at that point a call was placed. My father was taken by ambulance to the hospital, but by the time someone with severe hyperglycemia passes out, major damage likely has already been done. For Tom O'Connell, the damage was catastrophic.

Hearing my uncle recount this tragic tale brought to mind something my Aunt Auderie, a cheerleader on my father's high school basketball team, had told me over lunch at the Pennsauken Country Club. "Our generation, and the generations before us, were not people to run to the doctor," she said. "And as far as hospitals go—I know people who are the same way as your father. 'Oh, no,' they'd say. They hated going to the hospital to *visit* someone, let alone for themselves. They preferred denial: *If I don't go, then I won't get any bad news*, was their thinking."

WHEN I ARRIVE in L.A. for my second visit with my father, he looks far worse off than he did eighteen months earlier, when I last saw him. I've been told he hasn't been eating, and his body is now cadaverous. During my last visit, the stump remaining from his amputation had been covered; now it's exposed. The sight shouldn't surprise me, but I'm taken aback. His torso is covered with a polo shirt; his lower half, by a diaper. His remaining leg is propped up, and skinlike parchment flaps from the bone. His eyes widen when he sees me. Slowly, he extends an emaciated arm covered with blotches to hold my hand.

We don't speak much when I first arrive. It will take him several minutes to get his bearing and marshal his strength in the presence of a visitor, especially a son he hasn't seen in a year and a half, and for twenty years before that. I ask him if I can pull up a chair, and he nods yes while beginning the elaborate process of sitting up a bit in his bed.

His nurse Jennifer comes in and asks him to take a medication called Reglan. When a diabetic's nerve damage affects the stomach, a condition called diabetic gastroparesis, food just sits there because the muscles are no longer signaled to contract. The stomach is paralyzed. The resulting nausea, vomiting, heartburn, and fullness would kill anyone's appetite. Reglan is designed to increase stomach and small intestine contractions. In theory, this should aid with digestion, except my father can't swallow the pill and spits it back up. I pick up a washcloth from his tray table and gently wipe his mouth.

Neither one of us is a stellar conversationalist, but after a few minutes we begin talking to the extent that he is able to in this state.

"I'm sorry I haven't seen you since the last time," I say. "I really haven't flown anywhere for the last year because, frankly, I'm terrified of it."

"That makes two of us," he says with a slight grin.

"I've called a bunch of times, including Father's Day, but I always get the machine, and I haven't heard back."

"Yeah, I don't think it works anymore," he says.

"Still, I'm sorry it's been this long."

Normally this would be one of his better days, he says. There's no dialysis scheduled. But he says that he's feeling particularly under the weather today and dreading the prospect of having his blood cleaned again tomorrow.

For him to have survived for as long as he has, after what he's been through, is truly remarkable. "I'm not a quitter," whispers my father at one point. "I'd still like to have a few more good years." I suspect he has only a few weeks or months left, at the very most, but I tell him how great it will be when he leaves this place behind. He nods his head in agreement.

A month and a half earlier, he had suffered a seizure, which isn't unusual when diabetes advances to this stage. He'd been depressed ever since, I was told. That's typical, too.

MY FATHER SAYS that he needs a nap. I promise him I'll be here when he wakes up. When his eyes flutter back open after five minutes, he extends his arm for my hand, and we chat a little more. I tell him I'll be in L.A. for a few weeks and that I want to spend as much time with him as he can manage. I ask him if I can accompany him to a dialysis session. He's surprised but grants my request. "Nothing happens . . . it's really boring," he says. I tell him I'll bring reading material, and he manages a laugh.

The next morning, a pair of twenty-something paramedics, Kevin and Frederico, show up to transport my father to his dialysis session at another facility. "These guys are my buddies," my father says. Transferring his skeleton from hospital bed to gurney is a delicate dance. They end up grasping two corners each of the blanket underneath him, and then, on a synchronized count, lift him and the blanket from the bed to the gurney in one sweeping motion.

After my father's been wheeled out of the facility, one of the guys slides in behind the wheel of the ambulance. I pile into the back with my father, who remains on the gurney, and the other tech. During the fifteen-minute drive, Kevin explains that we're in a basic ambulance, lacking only drugs and a defibrillator. I ask him how many of their transports involve dialysis. He says 90 percent, noting that his company specializes in those calls. The business of kidney cleansing isn't cheap.

The two paramedics wheel my father into the Kidney Dialysis Center of Northridge. With stations arrayed around the large room, TVs hung from the ceiling, and technicians moving from person to person, it looks at first blush like a nail salon or Laundromat. Then I see that the frail, sickly bodies of patients, most of them elderly and swaddled in blankets, are hooked up to artificial kidneys. When the goal of diabetes care is simply to manage complications over time, rather than going to the source and addressing insulin resistance, this is where you wind up.

"I GUESS YOU know what's going on with your father," an angelic young technician named Sarah says to me. "Uh, sort of?" I reply, with more than a hint of embarrassment. I can't imagine the severe judgment she must be passing on a son who pleads ignorance when asked about his own father's suffering, which she witnesses several times a week. She fills me in on his weight loss and worsening mental outlook. What I didn't know was that my father had been cutting short his dialysis treatments. Whereas healthy kidneys work round the clock, dialysis has only twelve hours each week to attempt the same job. Shortchanging it will result in a dangerous nitrogen buildup in the blood and other harmful consequences. Given my father's frailty, I can't picture how he would stop a session even if he wanted to.

When Sarah leaves to tend to another patient, I turn to my father: "Dad, you have to try and make it through the whole session each time, okay? It's really important. You'll feel better if you can just do that."

They say children eventually become parents to their parents, but after such a long absence, I'm feeling woefully unqualified and unprepared for the job.

My father's father, the first Thomas Joseph O'Connell, also endured dialysis treatments until deciding that he would rather die than continue. "He asked me to meet him for a beer one day, and he said, 'I'm not going to do it anymore,'" my Uncle Hughie had told me the month before. "I said, 'Are you *sure* about this?' and he was." My grandfather, who I only met once or twice, perished within days. Eventually, many people would rather enact what amounts to a reverse assisted suicide than have their own blood being sent through the rinse cycle several times a week.

Kidney dialysis can be performed several ways, including an at-home version. My father is undergoing a technique called hemodialysis. Sarah tells me that she took up this occupation because her stepfather was a diabetic amputee who had to endure dialysis, and I can tell instantly that her empathy is great. She is as tender as one could be when inserting two catheters into my father's left arm, but his face screws into a mask of agony nonetheless. She has to connect the machine to his blood through a vein and artery that are his vascular "access portals"—a high volume of blood must travel through them each session. No wonder these thoroughfares look so sore and swollen.

"It doesn't hurt as much when they take them out," my father says as the pain subsides.

After spending three hours at the dialysis center, I realize the patient mix is more diverse than I had first thought. Many bundled-up bodies are wheeled in and out like my father's, but others come and go of their own accord, as if stopping by a tanning salon or dentist's office. A woman who looks to be in her forties approaches the exit holding a bag in each arm. I rise to open and hold the door, but she waves me off. "I do this all the time," she says. "I'm used to this baby. I leave dialysis and go party."

· · ·

AFTER WE RETURN to the care facility, and my father has been lifted back in his bed, he and I discuss our next visit. We plan it for two days hence. I hold his hand and tell him to sleep well, that I'll see him very soon. "Oh, call first," he says softly as I turn to leave. "I have this other family, and if you walk through the door when they're here, they'll be like, 'Whoa, who's this guy?'" He mimics a bewildered expression.

My father had always ignored the ripple effects of his decisions in life, and waiting until type 2 diabetes had devoured his right leg is just one recent example.

When I arrive on a Monday afternoon, I haven't called ahead, but he's expecting me. I can tell something is on his mind. I barely settle into a chair before he launches into a speech of sorts: "A long time ago, my wife and I decided to hide the fact from our kids that I had you kids from a previous marriage, to protect them. I remember it being her decision, and she says it was mine, but either way, it was a mistake."

"Protect them from *what?*" I snap. I'm a journalist. My older brother, the third Thomas Joseph O'Connell, is a Russia expert. My younger brother, a lawyer, is a vice president at a Los Angeles insurance company. No FBI-wanted poster material here.

He pauses but doesn't answer me. "She got very upset when that *Men's Health* article came out," he continued. "She said you weren't around for all that time and then you came back when you could make a buck. I told her, 'I don't know if that's true or not. I just want to spend some time with my son.'" As he finishes the sentence, his voice cracks and his eyes glisten.

"If you knew me, you would never think that," I say.

My father hesitates for a moment while searching my eyes. "But I don't know you."

When I had arrived three days earlier, he had mentioned how much he liked the *Men's Health* feature, how proud of me he was when reading it. As for not being around, well, my father vanished, not me. I wasn't the one hiding elements of my past.

He had reconnected with my two brothers sometime around 2000, but what I heard of those rare interactions sounded like a salt-soaked bandage being applied to an unhealed cut. My brothers would relate with bemusement how my father would pull out his wallet and display photos of his other kids. Who knows, maybe this was his awkward attempt at somehow trying to connect the dots of his lives into a coherent whole. Knowing my brothers, I'm sure they were just politely indulging their old man's eccentric obliviousness. I shook my head in disgust when I heard. *We know about them; they need to know about us*, I thought. *You've got this fucking backward.*

To me his outreach was moot because he still hadn't been sufficiently honest about who I was for reengagement to occur. His recognizing me fully and unconditionally as his son was a nonnegotiable prerequisite to any resumption of our relationship. That wouldn't change if type 2 diabetes had choked either one of us down to our next-to-the-last breath.

After my father finished his speech about his past mistakes, he fell silent. I went over and hugged him, kissed him on the forehead and cheek a few times, and said good-bye to him. I scribbled my number on a notepad and placed it on his tray table. "If anything changes, please give me a call," I said, turning to leave. "You know how I feel."

DIABETES REACHES A point where the victim's body can no longer be salvaged, and the same can be said of the ties that bind human beings, fathers and sons included. A shared disease, of all things, can't heal decades of neglect. Especially when the disease in question is itself borne of neglect. Perhaps subconsciously, I may have thought it could, and I was wrong. But my father and I were both wrong in thinking we didn't know each other. We knew each other better than either man would have ever cared to admit. When I walked out of his room that day, I would have bet my life that he would never pick up the phone and call the number I had left him. And he never did.

EPILOGUE

Two months after my last visit with my father, I spent Thanksgiving 2009 with my older brother, Tom, and his wife, Caroline, at their home in northern Virginia.

I sat in the living room with my mother's older sister, my Aunt Joan, whose homemade chocolate-chip cookies—the stuff of legend in my family—I had to decline after dinner. I watched a football game while she did needlepoint. She looked over.

"Your mother told me about your visit with your father," she said. "I'm sorry it didn't go well, hon."

We chatted about it, very briefly. I told her he was in bad shape and that he didn't have much time left. Before turning back to the game, I muttered, as much to myself as to her, "What's going to happen when he passes away? What, will there be, like, different funerals for each family?" The questions were rhetorical, needless to say. But an absurd situation leaves room for ridiculous contemplations.

My father was already dead, as it turned out. The next week my younger brother stopped by his care facility. The nurse said he had passed away a week and a half earlier.

MY FATHER'S LIFE served as a cautionary tale, all right, but not just about the perils of ignoring type 2 diabetes. Our parents influence us profoundly in childhood and adulthood alike, by positive and negative example. I will forever be indebted to my father for giving me plenty of both to draw upon in life. As for how long that life will last in light of my genetic predisposition to diabetes, I brim with optimism. The more disciplined and determined I become, the less concerned I am with measuring my blood sugar. I have a plan that works. What matters is doing what I need to do every day. When a nurse tested my fasting blood sugar in April 2010 using a finger prick and portable meter, which tend to produce higher readings than venous draws, the reading was 91, well within normal. I *never* thought I would get that low. But here I am, by most measures, metabolically mended.

In defiance of the myriad experts who believe in juggling carbs and drugs to address type 2 diabetes, I had wagered my future that clamping down hard on my carb intake while training every day was the only way to destroy type 2 diabetes. It's nearly four years later, and it seems I was right. You can achieve the same victory I did by following the steps outlined in this book. Once you decide that your heart, kidneys, and limbs are worth more than hamburger buns, french fries, and glazed doughnuts, you'll do more than avoid complications. You may find yourself in the best shape of your life. Don't think of this as the end of your best days; those are still coming your way.

One specter still loomed, though: the prospect of cardiovascular disease, given my family history of killer heart attacks and my prediabetes. That's the one mystery about my father's health that I could never crack. So much of his lineage had succumbed to heart failure; his own risk factors had been stratospheric for decades; and diabetes, which usually dooms the heart, had practically licked the flesh off of his bones. Yet as far I knew, his seventy-four years were devoid of a single cardiac "event." I couldn't help but think that the same ticker that had powered his storybook basketball season was the only thing willing that dismantled body to keep going. He lost his life to diabetes in the end, but I will say this about my father: He took this last opponent into an overtime period or two before finally surrendering.

In addition to my risk factors, the high-protein, high-fat diet I'd followed to combat diabetes is dismissed by the medical establishment precisely because they think it leads to heart disease. I had come to the conclusion that they were clueless and acted accordingly. Now it was time for me to put up or shut up.

I decided to have a test I had seen administered at the Amish Research Clinic in Lancaster County: an ultrasound of the carotid artery. As Patrick Donnelly, a research sonographer, had explained it to me during my visit, the carotid artery bifurcates before it enters the skull. Plaque will tend to accumulate where the blood eddies. If it does, chances are extraordinarily high that it's also accumulating in places nearer to the heart. The test is a great leading indicator of coronary artery disease.

If my test showed a lot of plaque, I'd not only have heart disease, but I'd also have to chuck my low-carb/high-fat anti-diabetes strategy. There was a lot at stake; this was a pivotal point in my life.

I've seldom felt as nervous as I did while the tech worked the wand up and down my neck. I heard strange sounds; his quizzical expression worried me. But as it turned out, the only strange thing about my ultrasound was that the blood kept shooting through the carotid so fast that he could barely do his readings, he said.

I asked him if he saw any plaque forming, like Donnelly had seen in the neck of Sally Fischer, the mother of fifteen. "I didn't see *any* plaque at all," he said. "And as fast as that blood is roaring through there—trust me, nothing's blocking that flow."

I was taken to another room, where the same sort of ultrasound test was to be done on the heart itself. Lying on my side in the glowing darkness, with a tech running the wand over my life source, I've seldom felt more helpless or vulnerable. I listened to several minutes of pumping and *whooshing* sounds, contemplating my own mortality all the while. I didn't know if these weird noises were promising or ominous, and the woman running the show from the chair beside me would play poker well. But for better or worse, this is the messy sound of human life, apparently.

An hour later the doctor came in with the results. "Wow, your echocardiogram is *awesome*," was the first thing she said, smiling.

I felt relief, and then I felt gratitude. A life-threatening disease wasn't the only thing my father had left me with, after all.

ACKNOWLEDGMENTS

To my late father, Thomas Joseph O'Connell, Jr., and my mother, Elaine Edythe O'Connell, thank you for the most generous of all gifts: life. I have never taken it for granted. Mom, thank you doubly for the support that gift came wrapped in. To my brothers, Tom and Marc O'Connell; and my two one-in-a-million sisters-in-law, Caroline O'Connell and Tanya Tan: I appreciate your love and encouragement.

I am indebted to Hughie O'Connell, not only for being the best uncle and godfather a guy could ever have, but also for filling in pieces of my father's past to which I wasn't privy. From submitting to hours of interviews to sweet-talking away the last remaining 1953 high school yearbook from a tenacious librarian named Edith Brown in Merchantville, New Jersey, he never failed to help me when asked, which was often.

Thanks to *Men's Health* for publishing "The Thin Man's Diabetes," which gave rise to this book; and "How Far Would You Go to Save Your Life?" a story idea that the magazine's deputy editor, Matt Marion, handed off to me. The reporting for both features informed my views on the intersection of genetics and lifestyle medicine. I still can't believe I actually have been paid to write for the magazine that would be my first choice off the magazine rack as a consumer.

The lightning-fast digits of Amel El-Zarou and Mindy Hantman transcribed the hundreds of interviews done for this book. Amel has been supplying my raw material from *A* to *Z* for a number of years. Her knowledge of blood sugar must surpass that of many doctors by now.

Over the years, many friends, acquaintances, and loved ones have taught me something that informs this work. I'm fortunate to have had such a grand cast inhabit the various stages of my life: Devin Alexander, my aunts Auderie (Moore) and Joan (Croasdale), Juliette Baez, Matt Bean, Cathy Clay, Jenna Bergen, Jeanine Detz, Karl-Edwin Guerre, Matt Goulding, Phil and Amy Jackson, Rita Madison, Rosanna Marshall, Melissa McNeese, Neena and Veena (aka Belly Twins), Megan Newman, Sherilee Newton, Natasha Pelak, Jimmy and Loretta Pena, Detective Ron Phillips, Jim Schmaltz, James Todd Smith (aka LL Cool J), and Zoraida Walker stand out among many more.

A special nod of appreciation goes to my hypnotherapist buddy Peter C. Siegel, R.P.H., who badgered me incessantly and supported me steadfastly until he passed away suddenly as I was writing this book. If heaven exists, I'm sure Pete's there now, sliding the pin into the bottom of the stack and hawking self-empowerment programs for the hereafter.

While researching a book like this one, a writer seeks information from many dozens of organizations. Invariably, a media-relations specialist or other point person fields and then directs the inquiry. These people are almost unfailingly helpful and receive little credit. Their names are too numerous to list, so I will thank them collectively. However, several went above and beyond to help me, especially John Webster, director of public and governmental affairs at the USDA Center for Nutrition Policy and Promotion; and Natasha M. McCoy, M.P.H., program manager for the Louisiana Diabetes Prevention and Control Program.

I'm indebted to the hundreds of experts who granted me interviews. Many of them are quoted herein; those who aren't informed its content nonetheless. These experts, most of whom handle Herculean work-loads at universities, share information with journalists like me because they think it might help people they don't even know. It's a sacrifice of their time and energy, and greatly appreciated.

I'm more deeply in hock to a smaller cadre of experts, some of whom became characters herein: Donald M. Barnett, M.D.; Jonny Bowden, C.N.S.; Barry Braun, Ph.D.; Harsh Doshi, M.D.; Joe Dowdell, a certi-fied strength and conditioning specialist; Cassandra Forsythe, Ph.D., R.D.; Chris Lockwood, Ph.D.; Christopher Mohr, Ph.D., R.D.; Ron Raab; Jeff Volek, Ph.D., R.D.; Jay Wortman, M.D.; Mary Vernon, M.D.; and Eric C. Westman, M.D. Each helped me when asked and as needed. The few who were acquaintances before my prediabetes diag-nosis encouraged me to call them out of the blue with questions (e.g, "Hey, can I order such and such with my steak?" Or, "What do you think of this workout I'm considering?"). Several others allowed me to enter their lives for a few days, introduced me to their diabetic patients, and placed their own work on hold until I had everything I needed.

I gained unique insights from a series of conference calls with my former Weider Publications colleagues James E. Wright, Ph.D., and Jeff Feliciano, who will always be the smartest guys in any room they oc-cupy. I've known Jim and Jeff since Jerry Kindela gave me my start in consumer magazines by hiring me as a copy editor at *Flex*, and I'm heartened that those bonds remain intact.

Of all the experts who helped me take my whacks into the Gordian knot that is type 2 diabetes, none deserves more thanks than Keith W. Berkowitz, M.D. Knowledge precedes power when it comes to one's health, and I could only fight back against this threat once Keith had identified the enemy lurking within me.

I met Keith through Adam Campbell, a *Men's Health* editor. Adam's terrific report "The Cure for Diabetes" became my personal call to arms, as well as a blueprint for my own "The Thin Man's Diabetes," which he then edited with care and skill. When that feature became the idea for this book, he helped me yet again, directing me to new re-search, forwarding contact information, and encouraging me.

By far the best decision I made on this project came early on, when

I recruited Jerilyn Covert, a Dickinson College graduate and *Men's Health* copy editor, to assist me with research, copy editing, and fact checking. I'm left wondering how any young woman could be so dependable, smart, indefatigable, lovely, professional, funny, and wise beyond her years. I'm not sure which proved more valuable, her editorial or moral support, but both were indispensable. I should also thank her fiancé, Joe DeRosa, for allowing this project to monopolize so many of her weekends for a year.

While Jerilyn tracked down studies and kept her eyes on the verb tenses and parentheses, Steven Stiefel read many chapters from a more contemplative distance. A writer himself, he's been my best friend for more than a decade, so who better to appraise copy that merged personal history with medical reporting. Steve may have missed his true calling, however. Discussing the passages about my family with him is the closest I've come to psychotherapy. If I can pull you off that surfboard, I owe you a glass at Vino the next time I'm in Los Angeles.

Helping to sculpt and guide this manuscript once it arrived at Hyperion was editorial assistant Kate L. Griffin. Editors offer suggestions on everything from story structure to individual sentences, but enthusiasm and encouragement can be the most coveted contribution of all. I'm lucky indeed to have been able to work with an editor so skillful on all counts.

Thank you to Elisabeth Dyssegaard, Hyperion's editor in chief, and Christine Pride, senior editor at Hyperion, for making invaluable contributions to the manuscript as it worked its way through the publishing process. I can't imagine having a more supportive editorial team behind my work from start to finish.

To the wonderful Brenda Copeland, former executive editor at Hyperion, thank you for believing in this work from the proposal through the completed manuscript and beyond. Without your guiding hand, inspiring attitude, and deft editorial touch, I doubt that this book would be what it became. I know for a fact that it wouldn't have been nearly as much fun to write.

Finally there is only the one person without whom this book would not exist—my agent, Marc Gerald, vice president and head of the literary department at The Agency Group. Marc saw the potential for my *Men's Health* feature to become a book before I did. My respect and appreciation for him as an advocate is surpassed only by my regard for him as a friend. Thank you for helping to shape my career with such enthusiasm, patience, and insight. Whether I'm winning a round or hitting the canvas with a thud, I know that you'll be in my corner when the bell rings.

NOTES

1: Ground Zero: Diabetes in the Delta

9   *What Is Type 2 Diabetes?* Sanofi-Aventis U.S. LLC (US.GLA.07.03.066, 2007).

10   *doubles the risk* T. Jeerakathil and others, "Short-Term Risk for Stroke Is Doubled in Persons with Newly Treated Type 2 Diabetes Compared with Persons Without Diabetes," *Stroke* 38 (2007): 1739–1743.

12   *The ADA's stated mission is to:* American Diabetes Association 69th Scientific Sessions, Final Program, front matter.

13   *reduced diabetes incidence:* Diabetes Prevention Program Research Group, "Reduction in the Incidence of Type 2 Diabetes with Lifestyle Intervention or Metformin," *New England Journal of Medicine* 346, no. 6 (February 7, 2002): 393–403.

2: Between the Devil and the DNA

29   *see their blemishes vanish:* R. N. Smith and others, "A Low-Glycemic-Load Diet Improves Symptoms in Acne Vulgaris Patients: a Randomized Controlled Trial," *American Journal of Clinical Nutrition* 86, no. 1 (2007): 107–15, accessed July 21, 2009, http://www.ajcn.org/cgi/content/full/86/1/107.

30   *men with thick hair*: M. Duskova and others, "What May Be the Markers of the
      Male Equivalent of Polycystic Ovary Syndrome?", *Physiological Research* 53
      (2004): 287–95.

30   *synonymous with insulin resistance*: L. Su and T. Chen, "Association of Androge-
      netic Alopecia with Metabolic Syndrome in Men: A Community-based Survey,"
      British Journal of Dermatology, 163, no. 2 (August 2010): 371–77.

34   *eating a carb-packed meal*: S. Nabb and D. Benton, "The Effect of the Interac-
      tion between Glucose Tolerance and Breakfasts Varying in Carbohydrate and
      Fibre on Mood and Cognition," *Nutritional Neuroscience* 9, nos. 3 and 4 (June
      2006): 161–8.

3: White Coats, White Flags

36   *has reached 26.8 million*: *IDF Diabetes Atlas*, 4th ed., International Diabetes
      Federation, 2009.

37   *prediabetic, a sugarcoated term*: "Number of People with Diabetes Increases to
      24 Million," Centers for Disease Control and Prevention, accessed August 30,
      2010, http://www.cdc.gov/media/pressrel/2008/r080624.htm.

38   *could remain ignorant*: "2007 National Diabetes Fact Sheet," Centers for Dis-
      ease Control and Prevention, accessed August 30, 2010. http://apps.nccd.cdc
      .gov/DDTSTRS/FactSheet.aspx.

38   *Seven years typically elapse*: C. D. Saudek and others, "A New Look at Screening
      and Diagnosing Diabetes Mellitus," *Journal of Clinical Endocrinology & Metabo-
      lism* 93, No. 7: 2447–53.

39   *hospital stays for diabetes*: Michael Corost, "Cost of Diabetes Drugs Soar,"
      HealthNewsDigest.com, October 30, 2008, accessed July 5, 2009, http://
      healthnewsdigest.com/news/Diabetes_Issues_640/Cost_of_Diabetes_Drugs_
      Soar.shtml.

40   *The World Health Organization expects*: "Diabetes Rates May Double World-
      wide by 2030," WebMD Health News Archive, accessed July 5, 2009, http://
      diabetes.webmd.com/news/20040426/diabetes-rates-worldwide.

42   *lacking many of the major risk factors*: R. Wildman and others, "The Obese with-
      out Cardiometabolic Risk Factor Clustering and the Normal Weight with Car-
      diometabolic Risk Factor Clustering," *Archives of Internal Medicine* 168, no. 15
      (2008): 1617–24.

42   *"metabolically benign obesity"*: S. Norbert and others, "Identification and Char-
      acterization of Metabolically Benign Obesity in Humans," *Archives of Internal
      Medicine* 168, no. 15 (2008): 1609–16.

43   *many fourth-year med students*: M. C. Lansang and H. Harrell, "Knowledge on
      Inpatient Diabetes among Fourth-Year Medical Students," *Diabetes Care* 30,

no. 5 (May 2007): 1088–91, accessed July 29, 2009, http://care.diabetesjournals.org/content/30/5/1088.full.

44   *missed at least half the time*: P. J. Leslie and others, "Hospital In-patient Statistics Underestimate the Morbidity Associated with Diabetes Mellitus," *Diabetic Medicine* 9 (1992): 379–85.

44   *their chart failed to mention*: C. S. Levetan and others, "Unrecognized Diabetes Among Hospitalized Patients," *Diabetes Care* 21 (1998): 246–9.

46   *The risk of diabetes was reduced*: J. Lindström and others, "The Finnish Diabetes Prevention Study (DPS): Lifestyle Intervention and 3-Year Results on Diet and Physical Activity," *Diabetes Care* 26, no. 12, 2003: 3230–6.

47   *"impact on physician career satisfaction"*: J. J. Stoddard and others, "Managed Care, Professional Autonomy, and Income: Effects on Physician Career Satisfaction," Abstract, *Journal of General Internal Medicine* 16 (October 2001): 675–84, accessed August 2, 2009, http://www.ncbi.nlm.nih.gov/pubmed/11679035.

51   *"Our medical establishment is set up to treat disease"*: J. O'Connell, "The Thin Man's Diabetes," *Men's Health* 23, no. 5 (May 2008): 160–68.

52   *"the patient should be carefully fed"*: Committee on Nutrition in Medical Education, Food and Nutrition Board, and National Research Council, *Nutrition Education in U.S. Medical Schools* (Washington D.C.: National Academy Press, 1985), 10.

53   *only 20 percent of U.S. medical schools*: Ibid.

53   *"future demands of the medical profession"*: Ibid.

54   *"and cultural diversity"*: Ibid.

54   *accredited U.S. medical schools*: Kelly M. Adams and others, "Status of Nutrition Education in Medical Schools," *American Journal of Clinical Nutrition* 83, no. 4 (2006): 941S–4S, accessed August 9, 2009, http://www.pubmedcentral.nih.gov/articlerender.fcgi?artid=2430660.

54   *"The amount of nutrition education"*: Ibid.

55   *The average American takes in*: Agricultural Research Service, "Products and Services," United States Department of Agriculture, accessed August 9, 2009, http://www.ars.usda.gov/Services/docs.htm?docid=17041.

57   *nutrition practice guidelines for adults*: American Dietetic Association, "ADA Diabetes Type 1 and 2 Evidence-based Nutrition Practice Guideline for Adults: Executive Summary of Guidelines," accessed August 9, 2009, http://www.adaevidencelibrary.com/topic.cfm?cat=3252&library=EBG.

4: Metabolic Mysteries

58   *more than half a million diabetics*: E. P. Joslin, "The Prevention of Diabetes Mellitus," *Journal of the American Medical Association* 76, no. 2 (January 8, 1921): 79–84.

58 *"odour of acetone to her breath"*: "Dr. Joslin's Magnificent Obsession," http://www.joslin.org/Files/EPJBiography.pdf.

60 *"tasted like honey, and was sticky to the touch"*: L. A. Witters and others, "Diabetes Detectives," *Dartmouth Medicine* 33, no. 2, (Winter 2008): 36–41, 56–7, accessed July 5, 2010, http://dartmed.dartmouth.edu/winter08/html/diabetes_detectives.php.

60 *type 1 children seldom lived for more than a year*: M. Sattley, "The History of Diabetes," *Diabetes Health* (November 1996), accessed September 10, 2010, http://www.diabeteshealth.com/read/2008/12/17/715/the-history-of-diabetes?section=203.

61 *like so many Florence Nightingales*: Ibid.

63 *This debate ended in 1993*: The Diabetes Control and Complications Trial Research Group, "The Effect of Intensive Treatment of Diabetes on the Development and Progression of Long-Term Complications in Insulin-Dependent Diabetes Mellitus," *New England Journal of Medicine* 329, no. 14 (September 30, 1993): 977–86.

67 *America's obesity and diabetes epidemics*: Supercourse, "Low Carbohydrate, Low Insulin, Moderate Protein, Healthy Fats as the Basis for Blood Glucose Normalization in Diabetes," University of Pittsburg, accessed August 24, 2009, http://www.pitt.edu/~super1/lecture/lec17721/index.htm R. Raab, "The Low-Carb Approach to Diabetes," Diabetes-Low-Carb, accessed August 24, 2009, http://www.diabetes-low-carb.org/.

68 *risk of developing type 2 diabetes dropped by 16 percent!*: R. F. Hamman, "Effect of Weight Loss with Lifestyle Intervention on Risk of Diabetes," *Diabetes Care* 29, no. 9 (2006): 2102–7.

69 *twice as likely as a white man*: M. Santora, "East Meets West: Adding Pounds and Peril," *New York Times*, January 12, 2006, accessed August 30, 2010, http://www.nytimes.com/2006/01/12/nyregion/nyregionspecial5/12diabetes.html?_r=2&hp&ex=1137128400&en=7a547abfaf515e29&ei=5094&partner=homepage.

71 *the U.S. spent $12.5 billion*: G. C. Alexander and others, "National Trends in Treatment of Type 2 Diabetes Mellitus, 1994–2007," *Archives of Internal Medicine* 168, no. 19 (2008): 2088–94.

71 *the global market for diabetes drugs*: D. Conover and K. Anderson, "The Broadening Spectrum of Diabetes Treatments," *Healthcare Observer* 3, no. 1 (August 2010): 1–41.

72 *tripled the number of carbs*: ADA.Macro.ppt, courtesy of the American Diabetes Association.

72 *"a stronger association has been observed"*: N. F. Sheard and others, "Dietary Carbohydrate (Amount and Type) in the Prevention and Management of Diabetes," *Diabetes Care* 27, no. 9 (September 2004): 2266–71.

73 *He called it Syndrome X*: G. M. Reaven, "Banting Lecture 1988. Role of Insulin Resistance in Human Disease," *Diabetes* 37 (1988): 1595–607, accessed August 29, 2009, http://www.ncbi.nlm.nih.gov/pubmed/3056758.

74 *European Group for the Study of Insulin Resistance*: "Research Activity of the EGIR Group," European Group for the Study of Insulin Resistance, accessed August 29, 2009, http://www.egir.org/load.php?menu=public&page=http:// www.egir.org/activity.html.

5: Come, Sweet Death

75 *saddled with another serious health problem*: "First-of-its-Kind National Report Reveals Estimated High Prevalence and Heavy Cost of Type 2 Diabetes Complications in America," Drugs.com, accessed August 29, 2009, http://www.drugs .com/clinical_trials/first-kind-national-report-reveals-estimated-prevalence -heavy-cost-type-2-diabetes-complications-519.html.

76 *only 4s and 5s to diabetes*: T. Parker-Pope, "Diabetes: Underrated, Insidious and Deadly," *New York Times*, July 1, 2008, accessed August 30, 2010, http://www .nytimes.com/2008/07/01/health/01well.html?_r=2&th=&adxnnl=1&oref= slogin&emc=th&adxnnlx=1214922665-wFmQQ367jinau/giI23Yzw&oref= slogin.

79 *boosts the odds for cancers*: F. Bravi and others, "Food Groups and Renal Cell Carcinoma: A Case-Control Study from Italy," *International Journal of Cancer* 120, no. 3 (2006): 681–5; P. Stattin and others, "Prospective Study of Hyperglycemia and Cancer Risk," *Diabetes Care* 30, no. 3 (March 2007): 561–7.

79 *twice as likely as others to suffer depression*: S. H. Golden and others, "Examining a Bidirectional Association Between Depressive Symptoms and Diabetes," *Journal of the American Medical Association* 299, no. 23 (2008): 2751–59.

80 *proteins that can wreck brain neurons*: L. Wood and S. Setter, "Type 3 Diabetes: Brain Diabetes?" *U.S. Pharmacist* 35, no. 5 (May 20, 2010): 36–41.

80 *the number one killer of Americans*: "Heart Disease Is the Number One Cause of Death," Centers for Disease Control and Prevention, accessed August 15, 2010, http://www.cdc.gov/DHDSP/announcements/american_heart_month.htm.

80 *susceptible to having these brain attacks*: D. Sander, K. Sander, and H. Poppert, "Review: Stroke in Type 2 Diabetes," *British Journal of Diabetes & Vascular Disease* 8, no. 5 (2008): 222–9, accessed August 29, 2009, http://dvd.sagepub.com/ cgi/content/refs/8/5/222.

80 *hypertension in the normal-weight and overweight*: S. M. Haffner and others, "Metabolic Precursors of Hypertension: The San Antonio Study," *Archives of Internal Medicine* 156 (1996): 1994–2001.

80 *linked insulin resistance with rheumatoid arthritis*: A. Rosenvinge and others,

"Insulin Resistance in Patients with Rheumatoid Arthritis: Effect of Anti-TNF Therapy," *Scandinavian Journal of Rheumatology* 36, no. 2 (2007): 91–6.

80 *other metabolic syndrome components*: P. H. Dessein, A. E. Stanwix, and B. I. Joffe, "Cardiovascular Risk in Rheumatoid Arthritis Versus Osteoarthritis: Acute Phase Response Related Decreased Insulin Sensitivity and High-Density Lipoprotein Cholesterol as well as Clustering of Metabolic Syndrome Features in Rheumatoid Arthritis," *Arthritis Research* 4 (2002): R5; P. H. Dessein and B. I. Joffe, "Insulin Resistance and Impaired Beta Cell Function in Rheumatoid Arthritis," *Arthritis & Rheumatism* 54, no. 9 (2006): 2765–75.

80 *arthritis sufferers*: "Mechanisms of Insulin Resistance in Persons with Rheumatoid Arthritis," DukeHealth.org, accessed August 29, 2009, http://www.duke health.org/clinicaltrials/20080815171551982?subject=Healthy%20Volunteers.

81 *second-leading cause of end-stage kidney disease*: "Kidney and Urologic Diseases Statistics for the United States," National Kidney and Urologic Diseases Information Clearinghouse, accessed August 29, 2009, http://kidney.niddk.nih.gov/kudiseases/pubs/kustats/.

81 *nonalcoholic fatty liver disease*: "Diabetes and Fatty Liver," MyDiabetesCentral.com, accessed August 29, 2009, http://www.healthcentral.com/diabetes/c/17/1363/fatty-liver.

81 *blindsided by cirrhosis or liver failure*: "Nonalcoholic Fatty Liver Disease," Mayo Clinic, accessed August 29, 2009, http://www.mayoclinic.com/health/nonalco holic-fatty-liver-disease/DS00577.

81 *raise the odds of liver disease*: "Diabetes: How Does It Affect My Liver?", Mayo Clinic, accessed August 29, 2009, http://www.mayoclinic.com/health/diabe tes/AN00193.

81 *double the risk of chronic liver disease*: American Gastroenterological Association, "Diabetes Doubles Risk of Liver Disease and Liver Cancer," *Medical News Today*, accessed August 29, 2009, http://www.medicalnewstoday.com/articles/5869.php.

81 *imagine living without eyesight*: "2007 National Diabetes Fact Sheet," Centers for Disease Control and Prevention, accessed August 29, 2009, http://apps.nccd.cdc.gov/DDTSTRS/FactSheet.aspx.

81 *the tiny blood vessels in the back of the eye*: "Facts about Diabetic Retinopathy," National Eye Institute, accessed August 29, 2009, http://www.nei.nih.gov/health/diabetic/retinopathy.asp.

81 *twelve thousand to twenty-four thousand people lose their sight*: "2007 National Diabetes Fact Sheet," Centers for Disease Control and Prevention, accessed August 29, 2009, http://apps.nccd.cdc.gov/DDTSTRS/FactSheet.aspx.

81 *blood vessels in the cochlea*: K. E. Bainbridge, H. J. Hoffman, and C. C. Cowie, "Diabetes and Hearing Impairment in the United States: Audiometric Evidence

from the National Health and Nutrition Examination Surveys, 1999 to 2004," *Annals of Internal Medicine* 149 (2008): 1–10.

81 *Those with periodontal disease*: R. T. Demmer, D. R. Jacobs, and M. Desvarieux, "Periodontal Disease and Incident Type 2 Diabetes: Results from the First National Health and Nutrition Examination Survey and its Epidemiologic Follow-Up Study," *Diabetes Care* 31, no. 7 (July 2008): 1373–9, accessed November 28, 2009, http://care.diabetesjournals.org/content/31/7.toc.

82 *This problem will strike*: "Erectile Dysfunction," National Kidney and Urologic Diseases Information Clearinghouse, accessed August 30, 2009, http://kidney .niddk.nih.gov/kudiseases/pubs/impotence/#cause.

82 *ten to fifteen years earlier in diabetics*: "Erectile Dysfunction (Impotence) and Diabetes," WebMD, accessed August 30, 2009, http://www.webmd.com/erec tile-dysfunction/guide/ed-diabetes.

82 *first your penis goes, then your heart*: H. Zheng and others, "Predictors for Erectile Dysfunction among Diabetics," *Diabetes Research and Clinical Practice* 71, no. 3 (2006): 313–9.

82 *short-circuit their orgasms*: J. Ramalho-Santos, S. Amaral, and P. J. Oliveira, "Diabetes and the Impairment of Reproductive Function: Possible Role of Mitochondria and Reactive Oxygen Species," *Current Diabetes Reviews* 4, no. 1: 46–54.

82 *increased difficulty conceiving*: B. Dokken, "How Does Diabetes Affect Female Fertility?", abcnews.com, November 12, 2007, accessed June 15, 2010, http:// abcnews.go.com/Health/DiabetesLivingWith/story?id=3813676.

82 *Five out of every thousand diabetics will experience an amputation*: e-mail message to author from Laura Zauderer, spokeswoman, Centers for Disease Control and Prevention, February 12, 2009.

83 *Prosthetics sales have nearly doubled*: D. Costello, "Soaring Diabetes Rates Wake Prosthetics Industry," *Los Angeles Times*, July 4, 2007, accessed August 30, 2009, http://articles.latimes.com/2007/jul/04/business/fi-limbs4.

83 *damages the DNA in a man's sperm*: I. M. Agbaje and others, "Insulin Dependant Diabetes Mellitus: Implications for Male Reproductive Function," *Human Reproduction* 22, no. 7 (July 2007): 1871–7.

83 *"This damage has a serious and detrimental effect"*: e-mail message to author from Con Mallidis, August 19, 2009.

83 *type 2 diabetes and sleep apnea seem to keep company*: E. Tasali, B. Mokhlesi, and E. Van Cauter, "Obstructive Sleep Apnea and Type 2 Diabetes: Interacting Epidemics," *Chest* 133, no. 2 (2008): 496–506.

83 *blood clots, a predictor of heart disease*: R. von Känel and others, "Association Between Polysomnographic Measures of Disrupted Sleep and Prothrombotic Factors," *Chest* 131 (2007): 733–9, accessed August 30, 2009, http://www .chestjournal.org/content/131/3/733.full.pdf.

85   *damage the inner walls of our arteries*: A. Ceriello, "Impaired Glucose Tolerance
     and Cardiovascular Disease: The Possible Role of Post-Prandial Hyperglycemia,"
     American Heart Journal 147, no. 5 (May 2004): 803–7.

86   *the greater the fluctuations, the more damage*: Poster 407 from 2009 American
     Diabetes Association conference book of abstracts.

86   *isn't a particularly reliable measure*: L. Henareh, M. Berglund, and S. Agewall,
     "Should Oral Glucose Tolerance Test Be a Routine Examination After a Myo-
     cardial Infarction?" *International Journal of Cardiology* 97 (2004): 21–4.

6: The Grave Consequence of Denial

89   *strike Indians at least ten to fifteen years earlier*: S. K. Bhargava and others, "Rela-
     tion of Serial Changes in Childhood Body-Mass Index to Impaired Glucose
     Tolerance in Young Adulthood," *New England Journal of Medicine* 350 (February
     26, 2004): 865–75.

90   *were all given a glucose tolerance test*: W. Yang and others, "Prevalence of Diabe-
     tes among Men and Women in China," *New England Journal of Medicine* 362,
     no. 12 (March 25, 2010): 1090–101.

91   *These numbers are climbing, too*: N. Duarte and others, "Obesity, Type II Diabe-
     tes and the Ala54Thr Polymorphism of Fatty Acid Binding Protein 2 in the
     Tongan Population," *Molecular Genetics and Metabolism* 79 (2003): 183–8.

92   *the First Nations' distant forebearers*: S. D. Phinney, J. A. Wortman, and D. Bibus,
     "Oolichan Grease: A Unique Marine Lipid and Dietary Staple of the North
     Pacific Coast," *Lipids* 44, no. 1 (January 2009): 47–51.

93   *wasn't even detected in Canada's aboriginals fifty years ago*: J. Reading, *The Crisis
     of Chronic Disease among Aboriginal Peoples: A Challenge for Public Health, Popula-
     tion Health, and Social Policy* (British Columbia, Canada: University of Victoria
     Centre for Aboriginal Health Research, 2009), 80.

96   *diets tended to include lots of protein*: L. Cordain and others, "Plant-Animal Sub-
     sistence Ratios and Macronutrient Energy Estimations in Worldwide Hunter-
     Gatherer Diets," *American Journal of Clinical Nutrition* 71, no. 3 (March 2000):
     682–92.

98   *Two groups falling below the mean*: "Number of People with Diabetes Increases
     to 24 Million," Centers for Disease Control and Prevention, press release, June
     2008, accessed October 18, 2009, http://www.cdc.gov/media/pressrel/2008/
     r080624.htm.

99   *men are slightly more likely than women to turn diabetic*: "2007 National Diabetes
     Fact Sheet," Centers for Disease Control and Prevention, accessed September
     22, 2010, http://www.cdc.gov/diabetes/pubs/pdf/ndfs_2007.pdf.

99   *"Genetic variation alone clearly cannot explain"*: S. O'Rahilly, "Science, Medicine,

and the Future Non-insulin Dependent Diabetes Mellitus: The Gathering Storm," *BMJ* 314 (March 29, 1997): 955, accessed October 10, 2009, http://www.bmj.com/cgi/content/full/314/7085/955.

99   *overfeeding of children*: M. Santora, "Bad Blood: East Meets West, Adding Pounds and Peril," *New York Times*, January 12, 2006, accessed October 18, 2009, http://www.nytimes.com/2006/01/12/nyregion/nyregionspecial5/12diabetes .html?_r=1&hp&ex=1137128400&en=7a547abfaf515e29&ei=5094&partner= homepage.

7: Reading Between the Lines

107   *"[Diabetes] pills work best"*: "Medication," American Diabetes Association, ac- cessed September 2, 2010, http://www.diabetes.org/type-2-diabetes/oral-medi cations.jsp.

108   *lower-than-normal testosterone levels*: S. Dhindsa and others, "Testosterone Con- centrations in Diabetic and Non-Diabetic Obese Men," *Diabetes Care* 33, no. 6 (June 2010): 1186–92.

109   *"we also let our members know"*: e-mail message to author from Leslie Champlin, public relations manager, American Academy of Family Physicians, May 22, 2009.

110   *"questions regarding the validity of recommendations"*: E. Nagy and others, "Do Guidelines for the Diagnosis and Monitoring of Diabetes Mellitus Fulfill the Criteria of Evidence-Based Guideline Development?", *Clinical Chemistry* 54 (2008): 1872–82.

110   *"The writings of the founders of modern medicine"*: N. Latov, "Evidence-Based Guidelines: Not Recommended," *Journal of American Physicians and Surgeons* 10, no. 1 (Spring 2005): 18–9.

111   *"We do not allow specific funding"*: e-mail message to author from Sue Kirkman, M.D., senior vice president of medical affairs and community information, American Diabetes Association, June 30, 2010.

112   *"some form of interaction"*: N. K. Choudry, H. T. Stelfox, and A. S. Detsky, "Relationships between Authors of Clinical Practice Guidelines and the Pharmaceutical Industry," *JAMA* 287 (2002): 612–7.

115   *echoed the thrust*: R. Taylor and J. Giles, "Cash Interests Taint Drug Advice," *Nature* 437 (October 20, 2005): 1070–1.

115   *conflicts of interest in clinical practice guidelines*: "Conflicts of Interest and Devel- opment of Clinical Practice Guidelines," in *Conflict of Interest in Medical Research, Education, and Practice*, eds. B. Lo and M.J. Field, (Washington, D.C: The National Academies Press, 2009), 189–215.

116   *recommended that metformin*: American Diabetes Association, "Standards of Dia- betic Care—2007," *Diabetes Care* 30, supplement no. 1 (January 2007): S4–S41.

116 *"Metformin is insurance"*: A. Campbell, "The Cure for Diabetes," *Men's Health* 21, no. 10 (December 2006): 136–42, 178.

116 *has only a slim chance of going off*: A. M. Emslie-Smith and others, "Contraindications to Metformin Therapy in Patients with Type 2 diabetes," *Diabetic Medicine* (June 2001): 483–8.

116 *"obese and under sixty years of age"*: D. M. Nathan and others, "Management of Hyperglycemia in Type 2 Diabetes: A Consensus Algorithm for the Initiation and Adjustment of Therapy: A Consensus Statement from the American Diabetes Association and the European Association for the Study of Diabetes," *Diabetes Care* 29, no. 8 (August 2006): 1963–72.

117 *decreased vitamin B12 absorption*: J. de Jager and others, "Long Term Treatment with Metformin in Patients with Type 2 Diabetes and Risk of Vitamin B-12 Deficiency: Randomised Placebo Controlled Trial," *BMJ* 340 (2010): c2181.

119 *exercise's beneficial effect waned*: unpublished data conveyed from Barry Braun to author by e-mail, August 4, 2009.

8: Prescriptions for a Disaster

121 *"to satisfy a gluttonous appetite"*: W. R. Campbell and J. J. R. Macleod, "Insulin," *Medicine* 3, no. 3 (August 1924): 195–308.

124 *"from an acute to a chronic disease"*: C. Feudtner, *Bittersweet: Diabetes, Insulin, and the Transformation of Illness* (Chapel Hill: The University of North Carolina Press, May 2003), 27.

124 *3.7 out of every thousand*: S. J. Kenny, R. E. Aubert, and L. Geiss, "Prevalence and Incidence of Non-insulin-dependent Diabetes," ed. M. Harris and others, *Diabetes in America* (Bethesda, Maryland: National Institutes of Health, 1995), 47–67.

124 *a $12.5-billion-in-sales market*: G. C. Alexander and others, "National Trends in Treatment of Type 2 Diabetes Mellitus, 1994–2007," *Archives of Internal Medicine* 168, no. 19 (October 27, 2008): 2088–94.

127 *"$6 billion pie to be carved up"*: S. Pettypiece, "Merck Diabetes Pill Januby Set to Rejuvenate Shares (Update 2)," Bloomberg, accessed August 11, 2010, http://www.bloomberg.com/apps/news?pid=20601103&sid=aIO._YCZ5Q24&refer=news.

127 *"Patients make less and less insulin"*: G. Kolata, "Looking Past Blood Sugar to Survive with Diabetes," *New York Times*, August 20, 2007, accessed November 18, 2009, http://www.nytimes.com/2007/08/20/health/20diabetes.html?pagewanted=1&_r=1.

128 *"Then we add a drug that stimulates that pancreas"*: Ibid.

128 *less than half the time*: G. C. Alexander and others, "National Trends in Treat-

ment of Type 2 Diabetes Mellitus, 1994–2007," *Archives of Internal Medicine* 168, no. 19 (October 27, 2008): 2088–94.

128 *diabetes drugs in a single product*: Ibid.

128 *the average cost of a diabetes prescription*: Ibid.

129 *more expensive diabetes drugs are no better*: Consumer Reports Best Buy Drugs, "Treating Type 2 Diabetes: The Oral Diabetes Drugs," accessed November 14, 2010, http://www.consumerreports.org/health/resources/pdf/best-buy-drugs/ DiabetesUpdate-FINAL-Feb09.pdf

129 *"The whole thing is crazy, it's shameful"*: R. Bernstein, podcast of interview on the low-carb diabetes solution, *The Livin' La Vida Low-Carb Show*, episode 264, accessed October 2, 2009, audiovisual file, http://www.thelivinlowcarbshow.com/ shownotes/288/dr-richard-bernstein-on-the-low-carb-diabetes-cure-ep-254/.

129 *twenty classes of drugs used to treat the fallout*: Jay Wortman, "The Poly-Pill Approach," Microsoft Powerpoint, e-mail attachment sent to author, September 10, 2009.

131 *enjoy some form of relationship*: E. G. Campbell and others, "A National Survey of Physician-Industry Relationships," *New England Journal of Medicine* 356 (2007): 1742–50.

134 *64 percent higher risk of a cardiovascular-related death*: S. E. Nissen and K. Wolski, "Effect of Rosiglitazone on the Risk of Myocardial Infarction and Death from Cardiovascular Causes," *New England Journal of Medicine* 356, no. 24 (June 14, 2007): 2457–1, accessed September 2, 2010, http://content.nejm.org/ cgi/content/abstract/356/24/2457.

134 *"contribute to adverse cardiovascular outcomes"*: Ibid.

134 *sales were down 27 percent*: J. DeHaven, "Diabetes Drug Poised to Boost Merck," *New Jersey Business News*, accessed October 4, 2009, http://www.nj.com/ business/index.ssf/2008/06/diabetes_drug_poised_to_boost.html.

135 *"mistakes that further obscured:"* G. Harris, "Diabetes Drug Maker Hid Test Data, Files Indicate," *New York Times*, published online July 12, 2010, accessed July 16, 2010, http://www.nytimes.com/2010/07/13/health/policy/13avandia .html.

136 *22 percent increase in deaths*: "NIH's ACCORD Clinical Trial Publishes Results: Researchers Still Have No Explanation for Deaths," American Academy of Family Physicians, July 2, 2008, accessed October 4, 2009, http://www.aafp. org/online/en/home/publications/news/news-now/clinical-care-research/ 20080702accord-results.html.

137 *A1C of the average U.S. type 2 diabetic*: W. T. Cefalu and K. Watson, "Intensive Glycemic Control and Cardiovascular Disease Observations From the ACCORD Study," *Diabetes* 57, no. 5 (May 2008): 1163–5, accessed October 14, 2009, http://diabetes.diabetesjournals.org/content/57/5/1163.full.

137 *hypoglycemic episodes, fluid retention*: "NIH's ACCORD Clinical Trial Publishes Results," American Academy of Family Physicians, July 2, 2008, accessed September 2, 2010, http://www.aafp.org/online/en/home/publications/news/news-now/clinical-care-research/20080702accord-results.html.

138 *difference in death rates*: "ACCORD Trial Mess," Weight of the Evidence, accessed October 4, 2009, http://weightoftheevidence.blogspot.com/2008/02/accord-trial-mess.html.

138 *compared to those taking oral meds*: C. Currie and others, "Survival as a Function of HbA1c in People with Type 2 Diabetes: A Retrospective Cohort Study," *Lancet* 375, no. 9713 (February 6, 2010): 481–9.

139 *our nation's first line of drug defense*: "Trends in the Prescribing of Thiazides for Hypertension," *PLoS Medicine* 2, no. 4 (April 2005): e113.

139 *The most effective of the three types*: "Choosing Blood Pressure Medications," Mayo Clinic, accessed September 2, 2010, http://www.mayoclinic.com/print/high-blood-pressure-medication/HI00028/METHOD=print.

139 *registered more than $42.5 million*: U.S. Bureau of the Census, *Current Industrial Reports*, "Pharmaceutical Preparations, Except Biologicals: 2005," June 2006, 3, http://www.census.gov/industry/1/ma325g05.pdf. ("Thiazides and related agents" is listed under the product code 325412D181.)

140 *negative effect of thiazides*: R. W. Wilkins, "New Drugs for the Treatment of Hypertension," *Annals of Internal Medicine* 5 (1959): 1–10.

140 *has been confirmed repeatedly*: P. J. Lewis and others, "Deterioration of Glucose Tolerance in Hypertensive Patients on Prolonged Diuretic Treatment," *Lancet* (March 13, 1976): 564–6.

140 *a review of fifty-nine relevant drug trials*: A. J. Zillich, "Thiazide Diuretics, Potassium, and the Development of Diabetes: A Quantitative Review," *Hypertension* 48, no. 2 (August 2006): 219–24.

140 *The thiazides make the beta cells*: H. A. Punzi, C. F. Punzi, and the Trinity Hypertension Research Institute, "Metabolic Issues in the Antihypertensive and Lipid-lowering Heart Attack Trial Study," *Current Hypertension Reports* 6 (2004): 106–10.

9: Putting the "Die" in Diet

143 *don't engage in enough activity*: D. R. Weiss and others, "Five-Year Predictors of Physical Activity Decline among Adults in Low-Income Communities: A Prospective Study," *International Journal of Behavioral Nutrition and Physical Activity* 4, no. 2 (2007), published online January 18, 2007, accessed on July 14, 2010, http://www.ncbi.nlm.nih.gov/pmc/articles/PMC1785385/.

145 *with an eye toward using subsidies*: D. E. Bowers, W. D. Rasmussen, and G. L.

Baker, *History of Agricultural Price-Support and Adjustment Programs, 1933–84.* United States Department of Agriculture, Economic Research Service, Agricultural Information Bulletin No. 485, 1984.

145   *22 percent of their disposable income on food*: B. Gardner, "U.S. Agriculture in the Twentieth Century," EH.Net Encyclopedia, ed. Robert Whaples, March 20, 2003, accessed on May 25, 2010, http://eh.net/encyclopedia/article/gardner .agriculture.us.

146   *The ADA's first diabetic diet*: E. K. Caso, "Calculation of Diabetic Diets," *Journal of the American Dietetic Association* 26 (1950): 575–83.

146   *frequent fast-food diners*: K. J. Duffey and others, "Regular Consumption from Fast Food Establishments Relative to other Restaurants is Differentially Associated with Metabolic Outcomes in Young Adults," *Journal of Nutrition* 139, no. 11 (November 2009): 2113–8; M. A. Pereira, "Fast-Food Habits, Weight Gain, and Insulin Resistance (the CARDIA study): 15-year Prospective Analysis," *Lancet* 365, no. 9453 (January 1–7): 36–42.

147   *"kills nearly everyone with diabetes"*: G. Kolata, "Looking Past Blood Sugar to Survive with Diabetes," *New York Times*, August 20, 2007, accessed November 16, 2009, http://www.nytimes.com/2007/08/20/health/20diabetes.html?page- wanted=1&_r=1.

148   *they recommended a seismic shift*: American Diabetes Association, "Nutritional Recommendations and Principles for Individuals with Diabetes Mellitus," *Diabetes Care* 10 (1987): 126–32.

149   *Wrote one of the Harvard experts*: W. C. Willett, *Eat, Drink, and Be Healthy: The Harvard Medical School Guide to Healthy Eating*, (New York, NY: Simon and Schuster), 2001, 16.

149   *The Harvard team designed their own version*: "What Should You Eat?" Harvard School of Public Health, accessed September 26, 2009, http://www.hsph.harvard .edu/nutritionsource/what-should-you-eat/pyramid/.

149   *MyPyramid, which debuted in 2005*: J. Lewis, "The Food Pyramid: Its History, Purpose, and Effectiveness," A 2 Z of Health, Beauty, and Fitness, accessed September 27, 2009, http://health.learninginfo.org/food-pyramid.htm.

150   *one in three U.S. adults . . . by 2050*: J. P. Boyle and others, "Projection of the Year 2050 Burden of Diabetes in the U.S. Adult Population: Dynamic Modeling of Incidence, Mortality, and Prediabetes Prevalence," *Population Health Metrics* vol. 8, no. 29 (October 22, 2010), accessed November 7, 2010, http://www.pophealth metrics.com/content/pdf/1478-7954-8-29.pdf.

152   *whose reduced-fat versions produce*: M. Fumento, "Busting the Low-Fat Dieting Myth," accessed September 27, 2009, http://www.fumento.com/fatlist.html.

152   *provided for the 2000 and 2005 guidelines*: United States Department of Agriculture, "Nutrition and Your Health: Dietary Guidelines for Americans," accessed

September 27, 2009, http://www.health.gov/dietaryguidelines/dga2005/comments/ViewAll.asp.

153 *"We see the value in collaborating"*: e-mail message to author from Colleen Fogarty, spokeswoman, American Diabetes Association, October 19, 2009.

155 *"nutrition assessment and treatment goals"*: American Diabetes Association, "Nutrition Recommendations and Principles for People with Diabetes Mellitus," *Diabetes Care* 17, no. 15 (May 1994): 519–22.

155 *to tame this metabolic beast*: American Diabetes Association, "Nutrition Recommendations and Interventions for Diabetes—2008," *Diabetes Care* 31, supplement no. 1 (2008): S61–S78.

157 *I like this breakdown*: R. D. Feinman, J. S. Volek, and E. C. Westman, "Dietary Carbohydrate Restriction in the Treatment of Diabetes and Metabolic Syndrome," *Clinical Nutrition Insight* 34, no. 12 (December 2008): 1–5.

158 *The losses are quicker and more pronounced*: K. J. Acheson, "Carbohydrate and Weight Control: Where Do We Stand?" *Current Opinion in Clinical Nutrition and Metabolic Care*, 7 (2004): 485–92.

158 *The research backs this up*: E. C. Westman, "Low Carbohydrate Nutrition and Metabolism," *American Journal of Clinical Nutrition* 86 (2007): 276–84.

160 *The need for diabetes meds goes away fast*: W. Yancy and others, "A Low-Carbohydrate, Ketogenic Diet to Treat Type 2 Diabetes," *Nutrition & Metabolism* 2 (2005): 34.

160 *apart from any loss of body weight*: M. C. Gannon and F. Q. Nuttall, "Control of Blood Glucose in Type 2 Diabetes without Weight Loss by Modification of Diet Composition," *Nutrition & Metabolism* 3, no. 16 (2006), accessed September 27, 2009, http://www.nutritionandmetabolism.com/content/3/1/16.

161 *a low-carb diet outperformed*: W. Yancy and others, "A Low-Carbohdyrate, Ketogenic Diet Versus a Low-Fat Diet to Treat Obesity and Hyperlipidemia," *Annals of Internal Medicine* 140 (2004): 769–77.

164 *measures of saturated fat in their blood went down*: J. S. Volek and others, "Carbohydrate Restriction Has a More Favorable Impact on the Metabolic Syndrome Than a Low Fat Diet," *Lipids* 44 (2009): 297–309.

165 *about twenty-six have focused on carbohydrates*: e-mail message to author from Colleen Fogarty, spokeswoman, American Diabetes Association, October 19, 2009.

10: Sweet Surrender

168 *the blood glucose concentration from a high-glycemic food*: D. S. Ludwig, "The Glycemic Index: Physiological Mechanisms Relating to Obesity, Diabetes, and Cardiovascular Disease," *JAMA* 287 (2002): 2414–23.

168 *consumed 600 to 700 more calories*: C. B. Ebbeling and others, "Effects of a Low-

Glycemic Load vs Low-Fat Diet in Obese Young Adults," *JAMA* 297, no. 19 (May 16, 2007): 2092–102, accessed November 11, 2009, http://jama.ama-assn .org/cgi/content/full/297/19/2092.

168 *cardiovascular disease*: S. Liu and others, "A Prospective Study of Dietary Glycemic Load, Carbohydrate Intake, and Risk of Coronary Heart Disease in U.S. Women," *American Journal of Clinical Nutrition* 71 (2000): 1455–61.

168 *cancer*: S. Franceschi and others, "Dietary Glycemic Load and Colorectal Cancer Risk," *Annals of Oncology* 12, no. 2 (February 2001): 173–8.

169 *divides the GI by 100*: J. Wylie-Rosett, C. J. Segal-Isaacson, and A. Segal-Isaacson, "Carbohydrates and Increases in Obesity: Does the Type of Carbohydrate Make a Difference?" *Obesity Research* 12 (2004): 124S–129S.

169 *they also upped their carb recommendations*: "Carbohydrates in Human Nutrition," Food and Agriculture Organization, accessed August 20, 2009, http:// www.fao.org/docrep/W8079E/w8079e00.htm.

169 *"these effects appear to be modest"*: M. J. Franz and others, "Evidence-Based Nutrition Principles and Recommendations for the Treatment and Prevention of Diabetes and Related Complications," *Diabetes Care* 25: 148–98, 2002.

169 *That stance was reiterated in a 2004 update*: American Diabetes Association, "Nutrition Principles and Recommendations in Diabetes (Position Statement), *Diabetes Care* 27, supplement 1 (2004): S36–S46.

169 *"provide a modest additional benefit"*: American Diabetes Association, "Nutrition Recommendations and Interventions for Diabetes—2008," *Diabetes Care* 31, supplement no. 1 (2008): S61–S78.

170 *This review looked at*: A. McGonigal and J. Kapustin, "Low-Glycemic Index Diets: Should They Be Recommended for Diabetics?" *Journal for Nurse Practitioners* 4, no. 9 (October 2008): 688–96.

171 *HFCS consumption in the United States increased tenfold*: "Fat of the Land: Do Agricultural Subsidies Foster Poor Health: HFCS: A Double-Edged Sword," MedScape Today, accessed August 23, 2009, http://www.medscape.com/view-article/491630_5.

171 *215 calories' worth per person per day*: "Sugar and Sweeteners: Recommended Data," United States Department of Agriculture, Economic Research Service, accessed September 2, 2010, http://www.ers.usda.gov/Briefing/Sugar/Data .htm. (Table 52 has data on HFCS consumption per capita, per year, from 1998 to 2008.)

172 *AGE formation accelerates*: M. Peppa, J. Uribarri, and H. Vlassara, "Glucose, Advanced Glycation End Products, and Diabetes Complications: What Is New and What Works," *Clinical Diabetes* 21, no. 4 (October 2003): 186–7, accessed September 2, 2010, http://clinical.diabetesjournals.org/cgi/content/full/21/4/ 186.

172 *metabolically active cells*: "Glycation," Chemistry Daily: The Chemistry Encyclopedia, accessed August 23, 2009, http://www.chemistrydaily.com/chemistry/
Glycation.

172 *Weakening of the collagen*: "What Are Advanced Glycation End Products?" Fitness Spotlight, accessed August 23, 2009, http://lifespotlight.com/health/2008/
12/01/what-are-advanced-glycation-end-products/.

173 *twenty-two teaspoons of added sugar a day*: R. K. Johnson and others, "Dietary
Sugars Intake and Cardiovascular Health: A Scientific Statement from the
American Heart Association," *Circulation*, published online before print, August 24, 2009, accessed August 25, 2009, http://circ.ahajournals.org/cgi/con
tent/abstract/CIRCULATIONAHA.108.838169v1].

173 *That's sixteen and thirteen more teaspoons*: Ibid.

173 *"HFCS didn't have the bad PR"*: e-mail message to author from Jonny Bowden,
July 9, 2009.

178 *healthy-heart benefits*: I. Shai and others, "Moderate Alcohol Intake and Markers
of Inflammation and Endothelial Dysfunction among Diabetic Men," *Diabetolo-
gia* 47, no. 10 (October 2004): 1760–7.

180 *a particular number of protein grams should produce*: N. W. Janney, "The Metabolic Relationship of the Proteins to Glucose," *Journal of Biological Chemistry*
20 (1915): 321–50.

180 *the fate of glucose*: P. A. Krezowski and others, "The Effect of Protein Ingestion
on the Metabolic Response to Oral Glucose in Normal Individuals," *American
Journal of Clinical Nutrition* 44 (1986): 847–56.

180 *might have been stored as glycogen*: e-mail and phone exchanges between author
and Mary C. Gannon, July 29, 2009.

180 *carb-induced rise in blood sugar*: From taped recording of lecture given at 2009
ADA conference: "Dietary Protein, Insulin Secretion and Diabetes," by Mary
C. Gannon.

182 *almost 20 percent less sugar*: G. Williams and others, "High Protein High Fibre
Snack Bars Reduce Food Intake and Improve Short Term Glucose and Insulin
Profiles Compared with High Fat Snack Bars," *Asia Pacific Journal of Clinical
Nutrition* 15, no. 4 (2006): 443–50.

183 *the effect pistachio nuts have*: "Eating Pistachios May Reduce the Impact of Carbohydrates on Blood Sugar Levels," *Medical News Today*, accessed August 23,
2009, https://www.medicalnewstoday.com/articles/69933.php.

183 *Jenkins and Kendall achieved similar results*: A. R. Josse and others, "Almonds
and Postprandial Glycemia—a Dose-Response Study," *Metabolism* 56, no. 3
(2007): 400–4.

183 *help offset the inflammatory response*: D. J. A. Jenkins and others, "Almonds De-

crease Postprandial Glycemia, Insulinemia, and Oxidative Damage in Healthy Individuals," *Journal of Nutrition*, 136 (December 2006): 2987–92.

186 *improves insulin sensitivity*: M. E. Rumawas and others, "Magnesium Intake Is Related to Improved Insulin Homeostasis in the Framingham Offspring Cohort," *Journal of the American College of Nutrition* 25, no. 6 (2006): 486–92.

189 *erythritol and mannitol*: Vickie Ewell, "The Truth About Sugar Alcohols," Kickin' Carb Clutter, accessed August 23, 2009, http://kickincarbclutter.blogspot.com/ 2007/08/truth-about-sugar-alcohols.html.

189 *maltitol provides enough glucose*: Ibid.

190 *those carbs are never subtracted*: Debby, September 4, 2003, comment on "What About Sugar Alcohols . . . Count Them or Not," http://www.atkinsdietbulletin-board.com/forums/atkins-low-carb-dieting-faqs/6731-what-about-sugar-alcohols -count-them-not.html.

190 *"it needs to be counted, period"*: Ibid.

11: Losing the Race to the Cure

194 *research team from Heriot-Watt University*: J. A. Babraj, "Extremely Short Duration High Intensity Interval Training Substantially Improves Insulin Action in Young Healthy Males," *BMC Endocrine Disorders* 9, no. 3 (January 2009), accessed August 2, 2009, http://www.pubmedcentral.nih.gov/articlerender.fcgi? tool=pubmed&pubmedid=19175906.

194 *their insulin resistance was improving*: B. Hendrick, "Brief, Rigorous Exercise Cuts Diabetes Risk," MedicineNet.com, accessed August 2, 2009, http://www .medicinenet.com/script/main/art.asp?articlekey=97212.

194 *I asked James Timmons*: e-mail messages to author from James Timmons, July 4–5, 2009.

195 *more intense training trumps more casual training*: A. E. Tjønna and others, "Aerobic Interval Training Versus Continuous Moderate Exercise as a Treatment for the Metabolic Syndrome," *Circulation* 118 no. 4 (2008): 346–54, published online before print July 7, 2008, accessed August 5, 2009, http://circ .ahajournals.org/cgi/content/abstract/118/4/346?maxtoshow=&HITS=10& hits=10&RESULTFORMAT=&fulltext=norway&searchid=1&FIRSTINDEX= 0&volume=118&issue=4&resourcetype=HWCIT.

195 *"guidelines are out of date"*: e-mail messages to author from James Timmons, July 4, 2009.

195 *"the behavior is reinforced"*: D. G. Marrero, "Time to Get Moving: Helping Patients with Diabetes Adopt Exercise as Part of a Healthy Lifestyle," *Clinical Diabetes* 23, no. 4 (October 2005): 154–9.

196   *regular exercise reduced diabetes incidence*: J. Tuomilehto and others, "Prevention of Type 2 Diabetes Mellitus by Changes in Lifestyle among Subjects with Impaired Glucose Tolerance," *New England Journal of Medicine* 344 (2001): 1343–50.

196   *44 percent reduction in diabetes risk*: L. A. Ahmad and J. P. Crandall, "Type 2 Diabetes Prevention: A Review," *Clinical Diabetes* 28, no. 2 (March 31, 2010): 53–9.

202   *the timing of that consumption*: B. R. Stephens and B. Braun, "Impact of Nutrient Intake Timing on the Metabolic Response to Exercise," *Nutrition Reviews* 66, no. 8 (2008): 473–6.

202   *the more carbs your body can absorb*: e-mail message to author from Barry Braun, August 7, 2009.

204   *the effect of exercise on this ratio*: K. J. Stewart and others, "Exercise Training Reverses Left Ventricular Diastolic Dysfunction in Type 2 Diabetes: A Randomized, Controlled Trial." Abstract, *Journal of Cardiopulmonary Rehabilitation and Prevention* 28 (2008): 271.

204   *three other diabetic-heart killers*: From taped recording of lecture given at 2009 ADA conference, Friday, June 5, 2009, "Reducing the Cardiovascular Consequences of Diabetes," Kerry J. Stewart, EdD.

205   *an excellent indicator of endothelial function*: A. Maiorana, "The Effect of Combined Aerobic and Resistance Exercise Training on Vascular Function in Type 2 Diabetes," *Journal of the American College of Cardiology* 38 (2001): 860–6.

206   *a joint position paper on diabetes and exercise*: American Diabetes Association/American College of Sports Medicine, "Diabetes Mellitus and Exercise," *Medicine & Science in Sports & Exercise* 29, no. 12 (December 1997): 1–6.

206   *ACSM released a new position stand*: American College of Sports Medicine, "Exercise and Type 2 Diabetes," *Medicine & Science in Sports & Exercise* 32, no. 7 (July 2000): 1345–60.

206   *the ADA revised its exercise recommendations*: American Diabetes Association, "Standards of Medical Care in Diabetes—2006," *Diabetes Care* 29, supplement no. 1 (January 2006): S4–S42.

207   *one night of partial sleep reduces insulin sensitivity*: E. Donga and others, "A Single Night of Partial Sleep Deprivation Induces Insulin Resistance in Multiple Metabolic Pathways in Healthy Subjects," *The Journal of Clinical Endocrinology & Metabolism*, 95, no. 6 (June 2010): 2963–8.

208   *"Restless Legs Syndrome and sleep apnea"*: R. C. Martins, M. L. Andersen, and S. Tufik, "The Reciprocal Interaction between Sleep and Type 2 Diabetes Mellitus: Facts and Perspectives," *Brazilian Journal of Medical and Biological Research* 41, no. 3 (March 2008): 180–7.

208   *Sleep apnea increases the risk*: E. Tasali and M. S. Ip, "Obstructive Sleep Apnea and Metabolic Syndrome: Alterations in Glucose Metabolism and Inflamma-

tion," *Proceedings of the American Thoracic Society* 5, no. 2 (February 15, 2008): 207–17.

12: A Sinking Feeling

217 *Your muscles start quaking*: "Nutrition for Reactive Hypoglycemia," McKinley Health Center at the University of Illinois at Urbana-Champaign, accessed July 13, 2009, http://www.mckinley.uiuc.edu/Handouts/hypoglycemia_nutrition_reactive.html.

221 *dipping into the guacamole*: http://www.sciencenews.org/view/generic/id/43015/title/Coming_Ersatz_calorie_restriction.

222 *caffeine heightens the perception*: J. Watson and D. Kerr, "The Best Defense Against Hypoglycemia Is to Recognize It: Is Caffeine Useful?" *Diabetes Technology & Therapeutics* 1, no. 2 (1999): 193–200.

223 *twice what the average American drinks*: National Coffee Association of U.S.A., *National Coffee Drinking Trends, Consumption Patterns from 1960 to Present* (New York, NY: National Coffee Association of U.S.A., 2000).

226 *We also become forgetful, anxious, aggressive*: "Hypoglycemia," University of Maryland Medical Center, accessed September 2, 2010, http://www.umm.edu/altmed/articles/hypoglycemia-000090.htm.

13: Barely a Shadow Cast

234 *Results take only five minutes*: e-mail message to author from Staci Gouveia, Bayer HealthCare, July 13, 2009.

235 *the ADA would amend its clinical practice guidelines*: American Diabetes Association, "Diagnosis and Classification of Diabetes Mellitus" (Position Statement), *Diabetes Care* 33, supplement 1: S62–S69.

238 *He received his medical degree in 1894*: "Honorees: Seale Harris, M.D.," Alabama Healthcare Hall of Fame, accessed July 13, 2009, http://www.healthcarehof.org/honorees99/harris.html.

239 *the solution for hyperinsulinism*: S. Harris, "The Diagnosis and Treatment of Hyperinsulinism," *Annals of Internal Medicine* 10, no. 4 (1936): 514–33.

239 *"landed on Dr. Harris like a ton of bricks"*: William Dufty, *Sugar Blues* (New York City: Grand Central, 1993), 82. (Paperback reprint of work originally published in 1975.)

240 *9,474 "refreshment places"*: U.S. Census Bureau, *Census of Retail Trade: Geographic Area Series—United States*, U.S. Department of Commerce Economics and Statistics Administration.

240 *registered $152 billion in sales*: U.S. Census Bureau, 2007 Economic Census.

240 *Minnesota Multiphasic Personality Inventory*: D. Anthony and others, "Personality Disorder and Reactive Hypoglycemia," *Diabetes* 22 (September 1973): 664–75.

240 *a forty-one-year-old veteran turned salesman*: C. T. Cerkez and K. G. Ferguson, "Diabetes Mellitus with Secondary Reactive Hypoglycemia Simulating a Neuropsychiatric Disorder," *Canadian Medical Association Journal* 92, no. 24 (June 12, 1965): 1270–3.

241 *when type 1 diabetic teens dip unaware*: K. S. Berlin and others, "Brief Report: Parent Perceptions of Hypoglycemic Symptoms of Youth with Diabetes; Disease Disclosure Minimizes Risk of Negative Evaluations," *Journal of Pediatric Psychology* 30, no. 2 (2005): 207–12.

242 *a 1971 issue of a journal*: J. H. Karam, "Reactive Hypoglycemia—Mechanisms and Management," *California Medicine* 114, no. 5 (May 1971): 64–70.

243 *journals and mainstream magazines*: E. Switzer, "Your Moods and Blood Sugar," *Vogue* (October 1973): 226.

243 *motor vehicle and washing-machine reviews*: "Low-blood Sugar: Fact or Fiction?" *Consumer Reports* 36 (1971): 444–6.

244 *Are the numbers for reactive hypoglycemia*: P. E. Cryer and others, "Evaluation and Management of Adult Hypoglycemic Disorders: An Endocrine Society Clinical Practice Guideline," *Journal of Clinical Endocrinology & Metabolism* 94 (2009): 709–28.

249 *"causes of most cases of reactive hypoglycemia"*: "Hypoglycemia," National Diabetes Information Clearinghouse, accessed September 2, 2010, http://diabetes.niddk.nih.gov/dm/pubs/hypoglycemia/.

249 *"recommend a diet high in protein"*: Ibid.

249 *While the sheet recommends protein foods*: Ibid.

250 *offers no clinical guidelines or policies*: e-mail message to author from Adam Lee, public relations specialist, American Academy of Family Physicians, August 14, 2009.

250 *"a clinical syndrome with diverse causes"*: F. J. Service, "Hypoglycemic Disorders," *New England Journal of Medicine* 332, no. 17 (April 27, 1995): 1144–52.

250 *"There's no discussion of reactive hypoglycemia"*: e-mail message to author from Eleese Cunningham, R.D., American Dietetic Association, August 18, 2009.

INDEX